A Gestalt Therapist's Guide Through the Depressive Field

This book is intended for psychotherapists working with depressed clients. In particular, it focuses on how working with depressed clients affects the therapists themselves, and elaborates on how therapists can care for themselves in such demanding work to prevent burnout, or process it meaningfully as part of their professional development.

Based on the results of the author's own long-term experience, qualitative research and theoretical concepts describing psychopathology from the humanistic-existential perspective of Gestalt therapy, this book describes a paradoxical way of working in which therapists transform their own experience in the presence of a depressed client. Using the example of working with depression, the book introduces how the field theory approach can be used in clinical practice. The book provides a conceptual framework, practical skills and case examples illustrating what a field theory approach brings to the table.

This will be a useful guide for psychotherapists and Gestalt therapists who regularly come into contact with depressive clients, as well as for therapists who are themselves experiencing professional exhaustion and are at risk of reaching burnout.

Jan Roubal, MD, PhD, is an associate professor at Masaryk University in Brno, Czech Republic, where he also works in the Center for Psychotherapy Research. He works as a psychotherapist and psychiatrist. He founded the Training in Psychotherapy Integration and the Training Gestalt Studia in the Czech Republic; he also works as a psychotherapy trainer and supervisor internationally.

The Gestalt Therapy Book Series

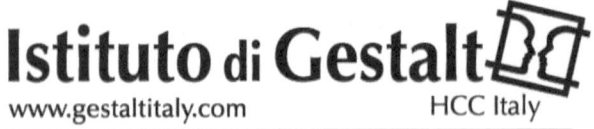

www.gestaltitaly.com   HCC Italy

Series Editor **Margherita Spagnuolo Lobb**

The Istituto di Gestalt series of Gestalt therapy books emerges from the ground of a growing interest in theory, research and clinical practice in the Gestalt community. The members of the Scientific and Editorial Boards have been committed for many years to the process of supporting research and publications in our field: through this series we want to offer our colleagues internationally the richness of the current trends in Gestalt therapy theory and practice, underpinned by research. The goal of this series is to develop the original principles in hermeneutic terms: to articulate a relational perspective, namely a phenomenological, aesthetic, field-oriented approach to psychotherapy. It is also intended to help professions and to support a solid development and dialogue of Gestalt therapy with other psychotherapeutic methods.

The series includes original books specifically created for it, as well as translations of volumes originally published in other languages. We hope that our editorial effort will support the growth of the Gestalt therapy community; a dialogue with other modalities and disciplines; and new developments in research, clinics and other fields where Gestalt therapy theory can be applied (e.g., organizations, education, political and social critique and movements).

We would like to dedicate this Gestalt Therapy Book Series to all our mentors and colleagues who have sown fruitful seeds in our minds and hearts.

Scientific Board
Vincent Béja, Dan Bloom, Bernd Bocian, Phil Brownell, Pietro A. Cavaleri, Scott Churchill, Michael Clemmens, Peter Cole, Susan L. Fischer, Madeleine Fogarty, Ruella Frank, Pablo Herrera Salinas, Lynne Jacobs, Natasha Kedrova, Timothy Leung, Alan Meara, Joseph Melnick, Myriam Muñoz Polit, Antonio Narzisi, Leanne O'Shea, Malcolm Parlett, Peter Philippson, Erving Polster, Jean-Marie Robine, Jan Roubal, Adriana Schnake, Peter Schulthess, Christine Stevens, Daan van Baalen, Carmen Vázquez Bandín, Gordon Wheeler, Gary Yontef

Editorial Board
Billy Desmond, Annette Hillers-Chen, Ann Kunish, Fabiola Maggio, Max Mishchenko, Georg Pernter, Rafael Salgado, Silvia Tosi, Jay Tropianskaia, Andy Williams, Jelena Zeleskov Djoric

"He calls this book, 'research' on therapy with depressive process. I prefer, 'communal lifeline.' Jan Roubal interviews himself and other therapists about our dark passages we must surrender to (not without a fight!), if we are to meet our severely depressed patients and find a way to walk with them toward the light. The stories move me, pain me and tell me I am not alone. Jan Roubal and his colleagues are now my communal lifeline in my work with severely depressed patients."

Lynne Jacobs, *Pacific Gestalt Institute*

"Among the many volumes on depression, this book is unique: rather than illustrating interventions on the patient, it is an exploration of how the therapist can inhabit depressive landscapes in order to modify the emerging dynamic. In this way, it is more than a text on how to do psychotherapy with a depressed client. It is a successful example of how to use field theory in clinical work: a revolution underway, though still in its beginning, in the world of psychotherapy and psychiatry."

Gianni Francesetti, *Turin School of Psychopathology,*
University of Turin

"I am delighted to commend this book on the difficult topic of working with depressed clients. Jan Roubal is a man who combines many qualities that make him a valuable guide in this field: professional skill as a psychiatrist, psychotherapist and trainer; honesty in his sharing of his processes; humanity and human care for his clients; and ability to combine theory and practice. This book is an illumination that helps us to enter this dark place safely and effectively."

Peter Philippson, *Manchester Gestalt Centre*

Coordinator
Stefania Benini

General Editor
Margherita Spagnuolo Lobb

Titles in the series:

For a full list of titles in this series, please visit www.routledge.com/Gestalt-Therapy/book-series/GESTHE and www.gestaltitaly.com

A Gestalt Therapist's Guide Through the Depressive Field

Giving Way to Hope

Jan Roubal

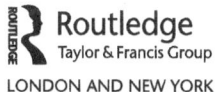
Routledge
Taylor & Francis Group

LONDON AND NEW YORK

Designed cover image: © Getty Images

First published in English 2025
by Routledge
4 Park Square, Milton Park, Abingdon, Oxon OX14 4RN

and by Routledge
605 Third Avenue, New York, NY 10158

Routledge is an imprint of the Taylor & Francis Group, an informa business

First published in Czech by Portál 2022

British Library Cataloguing-in-Publication Data
A catalogue record for this book is available from the British Library

Library of Congress Cataloging-in-Publication Data
Names: Roubal, Jan, 1971- author.
Title: A Gestalt therapist's guide through the depressive field : giving way to hope / Jan Roubal.
Description: Abingdon, Oxon ; New York, NY : Routledge, 2025. | Includes bibliographical references and index. |
Identifiers: LCCN 2024029210 (print) | LCCN 2024029211 (ebook) | ISBN 9781032814940 (paperback) | ISBN 9781032814957 (hardback) | ISBN 9781003500148 (ebook)
Subjects: MESH: Depressive Disorder--therapy | Gestalt Therapy | Psychotherapists--psychology | Burnout, Professional--prevention & control
Classification: LCC RC489.G4 R685 2025 (print) | LCC RC489.G4 (ebook) |
NLM WM 171.5 | DDC 616.89/143--dc23/eng/20240904
LC record available at https://lccn.loc.gov/2024029210
LC ebook record available at https://lccn.loc.gov/2024029211

ISBN: 978-1-032-81495-7 (hbk)
ISBN: 978-1-032-81494-0 (pbk)
ISBN: 978-1-003-50014-8 (ebk)

DOI: 10.4324/9781003500148

Typeset in Times New Roman
by KnowledgeWorks Global Ltd.

For everyone I have learned from along the way, with gratitude.

And for my wife Kristina, with love and thanks. For everything.

Contents

Acknowledgments

Additional funding from the Department of Psychology and Psychology Research Institute (Faculty of Social Studies, Masaryk University) is gratefully acknowledged.

Foreword

The struggle to overcome depression represents a major issue in the lives of many individuals and families in contemporary society. Depression can be experienced as an all-encompassing aspect of a person's way of being in the world, or it may accompany other life issues such as trauma or a medical condition. Depression can be both enduring and episodic. Psychotherapy is widely perceived as offering a potentially valuable means of moving beyond and coming to terms with depression. As a consequence, all counselors and psychotherapists encounter depression, and work with this condition – to a greater or lesser extent – in their routine practice. *A Gestalt Therapist's Guide Through the Depressive Field: Giving Way to Hope* makes an important contribution to a therapist's capacity to be responsive and helpful for clients for whom depression is a concern.

The starting point and primary focus of this book is on the lived experience of being a therapist working with a person who is depressed. A client who is in a depressed state is viewed as drawing their therapist into an emotional world characterized by hopelessness and despair. The central premise of this book is that any therapist – regardless of the theoretical model and techniques in which they have been trained – needs to be able to accept and handle their immersion in such an interpersonal field, in a way that allows them both to acknowledge the nature and depth of the client's suffering, and accompany them in their journey to a different position. Although the author draws on ideas from Gestalt therapy, psychoanalysis and neuroscience to make sense of aspects of this process, this book is essentially about the common ground of therapy, the threads of experience that are shared by all clients and therapists. It is therefore relevant for therapists of all backgrounds and theoretical orientations.

This is a carefully crafted book that operates at several levels. I am sure that different readers will find different things within it. I would like to briefly outline my own reader experience in relation to two key domains: research and practice.

The opening section of the book is anchored in an account of research carried out by the author into the experiences of therapists, from a range of therapy approaches, when working with depressed clients. Although I was already familiar with this program of research, in the form of published journal articles, it was enormously illuminating to be able to access a more relaxed, expansive and reflexive explanation of what motivated the author to conduct this research, its underlying conceptual rationale and its practical implications. Scientific articles in research journals tell a particular kind of story, that appropriately and necessarily highlights technical information about how a study was carried out and how it aligns with previous knowledge. By contrast, the early chapters of *Giving Way to Hope* tell a story about how an experienced therapist used research to deliberately get closer to aspects of their practice that troubled them, and how they were able to use this new understanding to enhance their awareness of what might be happening at points where therapy seemed to be stuck.

There is a lot in this book about what to do to facilitate learning and recovery in clients who are depressed. These ideas are formulated as general principles, of relevance to any approach to therapy, rather than as techniques or activities that are specific to a Gestalt orientation. One of these principles is to do one's best to grasp the client's experience, or the world they have created for themselves, as a whole. This helped me to realize that, like many therapists, I have had a tendency to want to find tangible therapeutic tasks that might enable a client to dismantle their depression, such as undoing self-critical thoughts, or activating behaviors that lead to pleasurable experiences and stronger connections with others. *Giving Way to Hope* suggests that, as well as these focused activities, it is important to work with a client to develop a shared understanding of the aesthetic quality of their overall way of being in the world. The idea of existing within a relational, embodied, social and temporal/historical *field*, that includes but also transcends one's personal sense of self, is proposed as a potentially useful means of gaining a perspective about one's world as a whole.

Alongside becoming more open to a big picture, *Giving Way to Hope* also advocates paying attention to small things that happen in the moment-by-moment experience of interacting therapeutically with a person who is depressed. The book includes several descriptions of micro-episodes in which a client said or did something in a session, the therapist had a visceral sense that what was happening was somehow new or significant, and then paused the flow of the session to stay with that moment and allow its meaning and significance to unfold. There is a very liberating dimension to how these events are described by the author as occurrences that are spontaneous, improvised and given, rather than being purposefully or consciously planned or constructed by either the client or therapist.

A further important practice principle that threads through this book is around sensitivity to metaphor as a means of conveying and reflecting on the quality of the client's experience as a whole. I will not spoil the reader's surprise and delight at encountering a core metaphor that is subtly introduced in the latter half of this book. Suffice to say that it is an image that is readily accessible and meaningful, that highlights the reality of being a person who is able to make choices but whose existence is shaped by forces beyond their control.

In addition to these – and other – principles for therapy for depression, *Giving Way to Hope* also includes sections that discuss the implications of an existential and relational approach to practical and ethical issues that arise in work with depressed clients, around such issues as the use of antidepressant medication, and suicidality.

This is a book that is based in showing as well as telling. The author uses case examples to show what working in a depressive field looks like in action. It is striking that, in these case vignettes, it is possible in every instance to understand how and why the client became depressed as a reaction to adverse circumstances in their life – there is no suggestion that their difficulties have been caused or exacerbated by any kind of chemical imbalance in their brain. A further characteristic of these case narratives is that they illustrate a therapy of humility, uncertainty and precarity. This is not a book in the tradition of entrepreneurial therapeutic triumphalism that characterizes so much of the contemporary literature. Instead, the author allows us to see his own personal self-doubt, and takes us with him on his continuing search to learn.

This is a challenging book that forcibly makes the point that therapists typically go through phases of withdrawing and turning away from their depressed clients, and invites the reader to look at their own practice from such a perspective. I warmly recommend this book to both trainee therapists and experienced practitioners. It offers an informative, stimulating and innovative exploration of what it is like to work with depressed clients, and how to use research to become a better therapist.

John McLeod
Institute for Integrative Counselling
and Psychotherapy, Dublin
Dundee, Scotland
April 2024

Introduction

I am writing this book for fatigued psychotherapists. For those of you who are sobering up after the first phase of beginner's enthusiasm or are even experiencing burnout. Through the example of working with patients suffering from depression, I try to show how psychotherapy can be dangerous for us therapists. Yet I also explore how we can meaningfully move through this dangerous field, and how there is joy to be found there.

Depression hurts immensely. As psychotherapists, we are tasked with trying to relieve the suffering of the depressed person. We sense their pain, we sympathize with them. But getting close to them in this way means immersing ourselves in their suffering; we have to "risk ourselves" (Rogers, in Anderson, 1997). Let me supplement this humanistic appeal with the instruction we hear before a flight: secure your own mask before helping others. In this book, I offer my perspective on how to put on such a mask in the psychotherapy of depression. As such, I do not write about how to work with depressed individuals. Rather, I address how to work with ourselves as therapists when we meet with someone else's depression.

Approved and recommended approaches for the psychotherapy of depression have been described many times. Instead of providing further appropriate therapeutic interventions, I would rather focus on an often neglected question: where do psychotherapeutic interventions come from? From what place does the therapist speak, in what way are they present? Even the most sophisticated and research-approved intervention will likely falter if carried out by a therapist who is also scared, unanchored, lost. On the other hand, even a completely ordinary and simple intervention, such as a smile, can do wonders. Such an intervention can be powerful if delivered by a therapist who is relaxed, grounded and personally attuned to their own intention in the here and now. And this is precisely what I want to get at: how can we as therapists work with ourselves? How can we set ourselves up to be truly present with a person who has sunk into the depths of depression?

The basic framework of my work is the humanistic-experiential approach of Gestalt therapy. It is my maternal psychotherapeutic language, so to speak, into which I integrate inspirations from elsewhere. I work in my own way, in which I feel grounded in myself, and I utilize that which I believe helps the people I work with. Similarly, this is how I try to present theoretical psychotherapeutic concepts

DOI: 10.4324/9781003500148-1

in this book. They are offered as inspiration for anyone to integrate into their own therapeutic approach.

Gestalt therapy is an approach that is based in the humanistic and existential tradition in psychotherapy. For me, this means that I try to see the client and myself in the uniqueness of our stories. To meet the client as another human being and be aware of the uniqueness of the moment. And also to humbly open myself to the unique process of meaning-making, in which, in that moment, the interweaving of our stories participates. It is meaning that transcends us and that we can experience through our physical presence here and now. I use the word unique here repeatedly because it represents a certain essence of this approach for me: what is happening now has never in history or anywhere in the world happened before nor will it ever or anywhere happen again. In my view, doing psychotherapy basically means returning to this simple principle repeatedly and experiencing it again and again when meeting another.

What I present in the forthcoming pages is a collage of practical experiences, theoretical concepts and research findings. Each of these components is written in a slightly different way. Notes from my practice are often quite simple ideas that help me in my work. Their simplicity is an advantage, because I can easily remember and hold on to them during a demanding moment with a client. I intertwine the practical experience with inspirations from theory and research. The selection of theoretical and research texts presented is highly subjective. I reference what reached me from theory, spoke to me and has helped me in my work.[1] I then supplement the practical and theoretical with the results of my research study on what happens to a psychotherapist who meets with a depressed client. How does the therapist experience this demanding situation, understand it and navigate it? What enables the therapist not only to cope with the situation, but then to potentially transform it?

In this book, I dare to present my understanding of concepts that I sometimes suspect I cannot fully understand. I consider the theoretical thinking of other authors and allow myself to borrow those aspects of their work that appeal to me and that coalesce in my mind in a way that helps me in my work. But I am painfully aware of how much I have not read about the experiences of others, how much I have missed from the accumulated wisdom of psychotherapists before me. At the same time, I suspect that reading it all would not rid me of the need to come to things for myself. And so I present to you what I have come to. And I hope that perhaps my text can serve as a reference point in your own theoretical thinking and help you go a little further in your own direction.

Before we delve further, I need to mention those without whom this book would not have come into being. Some parts of this book are my loose and revised adaptations of the texts I wrote with others. I try to distinguish the contributions of my colleagues with citations and primarily develop my own ideas here. In some instances, however, such a distinction is not entirely possible. Many ideas have grown out of our shared dialogue and are thus a joint work. Thus, with great gratitude, I would like to acknowledge the contributions of all my colleagues with whom I have grown during my professional journey and developed the various topics described in this book. I must specifically mention Gianni Francesetti (psychopathology, diagnostics, field theory), Michela Gecele (psychopathology, diagnostics), Elena Křivková (combination of psychotherapy and medication), Dave Mann (work with a suicidal client), Tomáš Řiháček (research project presented in this publication) and Stáňa Dudová (field theory). I am very grateful to all my colleagues who read this book in its rough draft and helped me chisel the final shape. I also think with gratitude about the people I met as clients and with whom I probably learned the most. You will meet some of them under the names Lucie, Richard, Daniel, Vojta, Monika, Valerie, Victor, Elisabeth, Michael and Susan.

I confess that I have one reckless ambition for this book: to outline how I imagine the practical application of field theory in psychotherapeutic work with people with psychopathological experiences, in this case depression. I attempt to describe how I view the depressive field. I examine it in detail as if under a magnifying glass, I hear it, I sense it. From various angles, I try to see what cannot be seen. To reveal what takes place yet does not materialize in a psychotherapeutic situation. To seek the source from where the observable phenomena of the psychotherapeutic process grows. In other words, I largely write about something that we can think of as a breeding ground or mycelium.

What I endeavor to write about here is the invisible mycelium of the here-and-now situation in which two people meet. I say little about depression itself and instead write more about the experiential background from which the mushroom[2] called depression grows. At the same time, I have a feeling that I will not be able to describe it, because words are too coarse and big for the fine filaments of the mycelium. By describing the ineffable delicateness and variability, I in fact destroy it. We cannot see the mycelium directly, it resides in the darkness underground. It is interconnected far more and spreads far beyond what we can imagine. I believe that this is what field theory tries to understand when describing processes at which I marvel, but cannot fully understand. Somehow, it even seems to be for my own good. My mind protects my mental health in this way and I am grateful to it for my obtuseness and limitedness.

As you can already tell, this may not be an easy read. It may take a second to tune in to my writing style, but please do. I write as if I am whittling a wood figure. I turn the wood over in my hand, carve off a flake, turn it again, shave off a bit elsewhere, then turn it back, and again and again. A shape gradually emerges. Likewise, throughout the following pages, I return to similar topics and shape them from different angles. I invite you on an adventure in search of a tangible shape that will begin to emerge. My intention, however, is not for you to eventually hold this shape firmly in your hands. Rather, I will try to help you tune into the fine fabric of the depressive mycelium. Using metaphors, stories and science, I hope to sensitize you to the mycelium of depression, to enable you to feel it when you meet with your client.

Essentially, I want to rid us therapists of the illusion that in our relation to a depressed person, we are not affected by their depression. It is my belief that in the presence of a depressed person, the depression grows through its mycelium into us as well. It thus affects how we are in contact with a depressed person. It probably cannot be any other way, nor would it make sense. After all, we need to risk ourselves to give the meeting with the depressed person a chance. Yet we as therapists can do this work consciously. By doing so, work in the depressive field can become a creative, enlivening and liberating process. Our freedom can then water the depressive mycelium. And we can watch what grows out of it. What happens to depression in a free and creative atmosphere?

Notes

1 This help has two forms for me. Firstly, theoretical concepts and research findings support me by allowing me to see my work as meaningful and embedded in a larger whole. Furthermore, they also arouse my curiosity, show me my routine work in a new light and perhaps partially protect me from burnout.
2 I use the mushroom metaphor repeatedly in this book. I consciously allow myself to ignore the fact that a fungus organism includes both an underground mycelium and an above-ground growth. For clarity of the metaphor, my terminology is that of a layman forest visitor. What can be seen growing above ground is what I call a mushroom.

Bibliography

Anderson, H. (1997). *Conversation, language, and possibilities: A postmodern approach to therapy*. Basic Books.
Eliot, T. S. (1943). *Four quartets*. Harcourt.

Chapter 1

How Depression Gets Under Our Skin

Lucie has struggled with depression repeatedly throughout her life. Irregularly and depending on specific events, she falls into a complete lack of energy, inactivity and disinterest for several months at a time. In the last three years, she has been hospitalized twice in a psychiatric ward. She has tried several antidepressants – "they help a little, not much." Lucie is 39, she lives in a village in a family house with her husband and two newly adult sons. She is on disability pension due to depression.

Lucie has been seeing me for psychotherapy for a year and a half. She likes the sessions, cries a lot and leaves feeling relaxed. "It's like an oasis here for me," she says. The surrounding world feels hostile and dangerous for her. She grew up in a family where her father beat her mother, drank heavily and humiliated everyone around him. She left home as soon as she could. Soon after she got married, her husband started drinking, beating her and humiliating her. Their sons learned to copy him. At home, everyone treats her "like a servant." For many years she has not really known anything else, and it won't get any better. She recently "accidentally" stepped off a moving train. She didn't want to kill herself, but she actually wouldn't mind being dead.

She inherited the house where she lives from her parents, but she does not have her own place there. At night, only when everyone goes to bed, she pushes the kitchen table aside and unfolds the sofa. In the morning, she has to put the kitchen back in order before the men get up. They scold her for being slow, stupid, "wrong in the head." She cries. "Don't bawl at us here. Save that for Roubal."

So I became part of the system. In our meetings "in the oasis" of psychotherapy, Lucie gathers strength to get through another week. In a week's time, she returns to psychotherapy, exhausted and beaten. I sit with her in that heaviness and hopelessness all over again. Relieved that she is not alone, she cries it out.

I like Lucie and I can't take much more of this anymore. What good is such psychotherapy? I am just helping to maintain the psychopathology of a family system. Hopelessness. That is what I experience with Lucie. And powerlessness. What needs to change, and how, is clear, but Lucie has neither the strength nor the courage to do it, and I have already tried everything I know. All I can do is offer her a safe place once a week where no one humiliates her. Where she

DOI: 10.4324/9781003500148-2

can gain some strength and then let herself be continually degraded and op-
pressed at home. A vicious circle. Powerlessness, hopelessness. Also fatigue,
exhaustion. And irritation, anger. I am being used as lubricant for the gears of a
pathological relationship machine. See you again next week, Lucie. Who's next?

At first, I noticed that I started to prefer writing notes rather than working directly with clients. It was less exhausting to sit alone, hidden away in my study at my computer, than to meet with the people who were waiting for my help. After five years of intensive psychotherapeutic work with depressed people, I didn't even want to see them anymore. It was an obligation I had to force myself into. Soon, my body started to reject it. In fact, I felt the reaction very physically. My body was refusing to sit in the therapy chair and it was making it very clear. Being with clients as a psychotherapist became a corporeal pain. When riding my bike after work, after kilometers of enjoying the exercise and the landscape, my clients' stories suddenly began to creep out of my body and into my mind. Suffering, pain, powerlessness and hopelessness seeped under my skin.

Then I became depressed myself. I remember the moment it dawned on me. I was supposed to catch a tram and even that ten-meter run was undoable, my legs were all water instead of muscle. I shuffled to the stop like an old man, the tram was already leaving and so I waited for the next. True burnout. I was forced to start taking care of myself. I'm not sure how much the actual antidepressants helped, but the important thing was admitting to myself that I couldn't manage this on my own. Psychotherapy helped me come to terms with reality. Not being alone in it all was key, as was redirecting my attention to taking care of my body and my spiritual world. I changed my job and reduced the number and severity of my clients. Gradually, that burnout experience became an important transformational milestone in my life. Not only personally, but also professionally.

I started to wonder what had actually happened to me. I had followed reasonable mental hygiene practices, separated my work from my personal life. My family life was happy and fulfilling, as was my time with friends and in pursuit of various interests. And yet depression got under my skin. It was as if I had soaked up the suffering of the people I met at work. As if I had been infected.

So I started to research what happened. I discovered that I was far from alone, that many of my colleagues had similar experiences, they were just not talking about it much. I also discovered that the "contagiousness of depression" is a phenomenon that has been studied for a relatively long time. And so I started investigating what happens to a therapist in contact with a depressed person.

My personal experience led me not only to this research, but also to theoretical thinking about the psychotherapy of depression. The turning point came when my burnout was at its peak. My wife and I were hiking high in the Alps. At the time, I was dragging my feet more than hiking, my mind busy with itself rather than taking in the surroundings. I walked a little off the track, facing a deep, rocky valley, into which my frustration suddenly screamed: "I don't want to fucking help anyone anymore!" It was a powerful moment, in which I perhaps broke out of the habitual way of relating to suffering that had been passed down from generation to generation for us. And it was also a strong professional impulse. I wanted to continue doing psychotherapy and yet I did not want to help anymore. Was it possible? What would I do with clients? And what good would it do them? It became a sort of koan for me and an intellectual challenge at the same time, which eventually led to this book.

Research Study: The Experience of Therapists During Psychotherapy Sessions with Depressed Clients

What happens to a psychotherapist in contact with a depressed client?[1] I decided to do more research on a topic that had affected me firsthand. Initially, I submerged myself into existing research findings. It was interesting to discover that what happens in our practice also happens in regard to the literature. We try to help the depressed person in front of us, yet forget about ourselves. There is a large body of clinical and research literature on how psychotherapy can help the client, but relatively little is known about the helper, who again and again encounters the emotionally demanding depressive states of their clients.

Noise in the Receiver

Unpleasant experiences with difficult clients represent a risk factor for the development of professional discomfort and burnout (Jenaro et al., 2007). Yet, psychotherapists generally tend to discount such experiences with clients as random and purely subjective, or even devalue them as inconvenient, counterproductive, and unprofessional (Wolf et al., 2013). By perceiving their own reactions only as "noise" in the psychotherapeutic process, psychotherapists not only increase the risk of developing burnout, but also "risk losing an important source of data that can directly or indirectly affect the psychotherapeutic alliance and have a negative effect on treatment outcomes" (Wolf et al., 2013, p. 8). Ignoring psychotherapists' own experiential responses can even lead to harming the client (Castonguay, Boswell, Constantino, Goldfried & Hill, 2010).

The experiences of therapists are still a relatively neglected area of research. Authorities in the profession (Najavits, 2000; Hayes & Gelso, 2001) therefore emphasize the importance of addressing them as significant clinical phenomena that naturally occur in everyday practice and that psychotherapists can use to enhance the therapeutic process. Specifically with depressed clients, it is especially crucial to investigate those interactions in which the depressed person is rejected by others (Gurtman, 1986).

We can deduce a lot about the effect of depression on the therapist from interpersonal theories of depression, which elaborate on how depression develops and is maintained in relationships. We can assume that these relational aspects also appear in the psychotherapeutic relationship, where it is likewise possible to address them. Nevertheless, research on how psychotherapeutic work with depression affects therapists is direly lacking. Researchers limit themselves to enumerating therapists' experiences with depressed clients and on occasion comparing them to therapists' responses to clients with other diagnoses, such as schizophrenic or borderline personality disorders (Boswell & Murray, 1981; Brody & Farber, 1996; McIntyre & Schwartz, 1998).

There is also little differentiation between the long-term effects and the immediate effect of depression directly during the session. Although some studies have examined therapists' experiences during sessions (e.g., Deutsch, 1984; Howard, Orlinsky & Hill, 1969; Williams, Polster, Grizzard, Rockenbaugh & Judge, 2003), they have done so in a general way and not specific to the therapy of depression.

For my qualitative research study, I chose the research question: *"How do therapists experience a psychotherapy session with a currently depressed client?"* I turned to my colleagues. First, I conducted semi-structured individual interviews with therapists who work with depressed clients. We explored their experiences in depth. I asked them:

"How do you recall your psychotherapy session with a client who is currently depressed?"
"What did you experience during this session?"
"How did your experience evolve?"
"What did you do?"
"What helped you?"
"What happened after?"
"Can you think of an apt metaphor for what happened in the session?"

Based on these interviews, I created a provisional theoretical model, which we further developed during discussions in groups of other therapists.[2]

What Experiences Does Depression Induce in a Therapist?

When analyzing the interviews, I focused on the experiences of the therapists, which they themselves attributed to their respective client's depressive state during the psychotherapy sessions. I left aside the other experiences of the therapists, namely the therapists' personal reactions to the client's personality or their life story and how these related to the therapist's own history, to their own processes.

I found justification for such a division in the literature as well. Therapists' experiences with clients have generally been theoretically incorporated into the concept of countertransference. This concept has undergone a long and complex development. In general, mainstream theories today consider countertransference as a phenomenon related to feelings and emotions that is co-constructed by both client and therapist (Gabbard, 1999). In their integrative concept, Gelso and Hayes (2007) divided therapists' subjective experiences into (1) a countertransference component associated with the therapist's personal unresolved conflicts and vulnerabilities, and (2) a non-countertransference component that includes the therapist's reactions triggered by the client's condition or behavior.

My research focuses on this second component. I am referring to Winnicott's (1949) somewhat older concept of "objective" countertransference, which involves generally human reactions to the client's specific ways of relating. I also refer to the examination of therapists' reactions to the characteristic ways in which clients evoke reactions in others (Homqvist & Armelius, 1996) or to the description of the therapist's "situational" difficulties (Schröder & Davis, 2004).

I am grateful for the trust of my colleagues, who were willing to talk to me very openly. They often described experiences of which they were a little ashamed and that they usually kept to themselves. Yet there was also a certain thrill of discovery in the interviews, as we uncovered the deeper layers and subtler nuances of what they experience with depressed clients.

I subsequently processed the interviews using the qualitative research method of grounded theory. This enables a detailed understanding of the investigated process. The end result of grounded theory is usually a compact and simple model of "how things work" in a certain defined area (Glaser & Strauss, 1967; Strauss & Corbin, 1990; Charmaz, 2006).[3]

I found that in psychotherapy sessions, "things work" roughly like this: Psychotherapists seem to experientially move in two opposite directions – they move closer to depression, or on the contrary, further away from it. In this way, during a session, they continuously "approach" and "distance" themselves from the depressed client. One of the therapists described it metaphorically as a movement up and down in a well:

The well is like the depth of the depression and (...) the surface is the daylight. (...) And I either let go of the client and get mad at them, or I let go of the surface and be there with [the client] and start to identify with them. (...) [The surface] is the daily reality. The way I normally am, living in my own world.

The Polarized Experiences of Psychotherapists

The presence of a depressed person generally causes two basic reactions in people (Coyne, 1976): they begin to feel depressed themselves, or they reject the depressed person. Psychotherapists are no different. When working with clients with treatment-resistant depression, they experience a wide range of emotions (McPherson, Walker & Carlyle, 2006; Levenson, 2013), from caring reactions (feelings of closeness, understanding or concern) to intensely unpleasant reactions (feelings of powerlessness, failure, incompetence, exhaustion, despondency, frustration or distress). "On the one hand, the psychotherapist feels rejected by the client and paralyzed by the depressive symptomatology, which often results in the psychotherapist's aggressiveness towards the client (...). On the other hand, depressed clients elicit a great deal of care, which can very quickly lead to extreme care or control over the client" (Rahn & Mahnkopf, 1999, p. 242).

Psychotherapists experience a fundamental tension between their professional attitude and their personal emotional response to a suffering person. A number of studies have repeatedly shown that depressed people elicit a dismissive or even hostile response from others (e.g., Gotlib & Robinson, 1982; Gurtman et al., 1990; Marks & Hammen, 1982; Paukert, Pettit & Amacker, 2008; Strack & Coyne, 1983; Winer, Bonner, Blaney & Murray, 1981). The psychotherapist's human reaction (frustration, boredom, fear, anger, hatred) can then be understood as "forces that pull the psychotherapist away from his professional ideal" (Wolf et al., 2013, p. 4). The therapist's experiential distancing from the client seems to be an automatic response to the depressing and exhausting feelings that a depressed client generally evokes in others.

From the perspective of psychoanalysis (McWilliams, 2011, p. 250), the therapist's experience with a depressed client can be understood as two opposing reactions: the psychotherapist either envisions being "the sensitive, accepting parent the client never had," or, on the contrary, may feel "incompetent, flawed, damaging, 'not good enough' (introjective elements) or desperate, demoralized and useless (anaclitic elements)." The therapist may then view their own anger as an indicator of their unfulfilled needs in the therapeutic relationship, and may see their own hatred as the force enabling them to break free from the burden of their unfulfilled needs (Green, 2006). It appears that the therapist's own unfulfilled needs combined with the client's excessive reassurance-seeking, which is specific to depression (Joiner, Metalsky, Gencoz & Gencoz, 2001), result in the therapist's detached experiential response.

Thus, the therapist's experiences oscillate between *sharing the depressive experience* and *distancing from the depressive experience* and gradually develop during the psychotherapy session. We explored this process in detail. The result is a general model of the *Trajectory of co-experiencing depression* (Roubal & Řiháček, 2016), which distinguishes the individual phases of this trajectory and their typical sequence. This model will be presented in Chapter 4, "Therapists in the Depressive Swamp." With the help of such a model, we can follow the changes in the experiences of psychotherapists, name the relationships between different experiences and relate them to other processes taking place during psychotherapy sessions.[4]

Notes

1 Due to my focus on the therapist, I avoid a more detailed classification of depressive experiences. Instead, I leave room for each therapist-reader to apply the finer nuances of how they themselves experientially resonate with the specific depression of their particular client.

2 In total, 30 psychotherapists participated in the research, of which 17 were women and 13 were men. Their theoretical orientations were: dynamic and psychoanalytic psychotherapy (16), humanistic/experiential/phenomenological psychotherapy (15), family/systemic therapy (3), integrative psychotherapy (2), and cognitive behavioral therapy (2). Of these, 23 therapists completed 1 psychotherapy training, 6 therapists completed 2 trainings and 1 therapist completed 3 trainings.

3 For a detailed analysis of the method used, see *An adventure in grounded theory method: Discovering a pattern in the flow of a therapy process* (Roubal & Řiháček, 2016).

4 Before we delve further into the experiences of therapists when meeting with depressed clients, some of you might want to stop and consider the very beginning of such an encounter. The moment we as therapists realize: this person is depressed. What happens to our attitude toward the client at that moment, what demands do we implicitly place on ourselves? How do we define the space where the psychotherapy process can go? If you are interested in this, see Chapter 12 at the end of the book, where I elaborate on how to use diagnosis to support the psychotherapy process.

Bibliography

Boswell, P. C., & Murray, E. J. (1981). Depression, schizophrenia and social attraction. *Journal of Consulting and Clinical Psychology*, *49*(5), 641–647.

Brody, E. M., & Farber, B. A. (1996). The effects of therapist experience and patient diagnosis on countertransference. *Psychotherapy*, 33(3), 372–380.

Burton, R. (2021). *The anatomy of melancholy*. Penguin Classics, p. 31.

Castonguay, L. G., Boswell, J. F., Constantino, M. J., Goldfried, M. R., Hill, C. E. (2010). Training implications of harmful effects of psychological treatments. *American Psychologist*, 65, 34–49.

Charmaz, K. (2006). *Constructing grounded theory: A practical guide through qualitative analysis*. Sage.

Coyne, J. C. (1976). Toward an interactional description of depression. *Psychiatry*, 39, 28–40.

Deutsch, C. J. (1984). Self-reported sources of stress among psychotherapists. *Professional Psychology: Research and Practice*, 15(6), 833–845.

Gabbard, G. O. (1999). *Countertransference issues in psychiatric treatment.* American Psychiatric Press.

Gelso, C. J., Hayes, J. A. (2007). *Countertransference and the therapist's inner experience: Perils and possibilities.* Lawrence Erlbaum Associates.

Glaser, B. G., Strauss, A. L. (1967). *The discovery of grounded theory: Strategies for qualitative research.* Aldine.

Gotlib, I. H., Robinson, L. A. (1982). Response to depressed individuals: Discrepancies between self-report and observer-rated behavior. *Journal of Abnormal Psychology, 91,* 231–240.

Green, L. B. (2006). The value of hate in the countertransference. *Clinical Social Work Journal, 34*(2), 187–199.

Gurtman, M. B. (1986). Depression and the response of others: Reevaluating the reevaluation. *Journal of Abnormal Psychology, 95*(1), 99–101.

Gurtman, M. B., Martin, K. M., & Hintzman, N. M. (1990). Interpersonal reactions to displays of depression and anxiety. *Journal of Social and Clinical Psychology, 9,* 256–267.

Hayes, J. A., & Gelso, C. J. (2001). Clinical implications of research on countertransference: Science informing practice. *Psychotherapy in Practice, 57*(8), 1041–1051.

Homqvist, R., Armelius, B. (1996). Sources of therapists' countertransference feelings. *Psychotherapy Research, 6,* 70–78.

Howard, K. I., Orlinsky, D. E., & Hill, J. A. (1969). The therapist's feelings in the therapeutic process. *Journal of Clinical Psychology, 25*(1), 83–93.

Jenaro, C., Flores, N., Arias, B. (2007). Burnout and coping in human service practitioners. *Professional Psychology: Research and Practice, 38,* 80–87.

Joiner, T. E., Metalsky, G. I., Gencoz, F., Gencoz, T. (2001). The relative specificity of excessive reassurance-seeking to depressive symptoms and diagnoses among clinical samples of adults and youth. *Journal of Psychopathology and Behavioral Assessment, 23*(1), 35–41.

Levenson, H. (2013). Time-limited dynamic psychotherapy: Working with reactions to chronically depressed clients. In Wolf, A. W., Goldfried, M. R., Muran, J. C (Eds.), *Transforming negative reactions to clients: From frustration to compassion.* American Psychological Association, 191–219.

Marks, T., Hammen, C. L. (1982). Interpersonal mood induction: Situational and individual determinants. *Motivation and Emotion, 6,* 387–399.

McIntyre, M. S., & Schwartz, R. C. (1998). Therapists' differential countertransference reactions toward clients with major depression or borderline personality disorder. *Journal of Clinical Psychology, 54*(7), 923–931.

McPherson, S., Walker, C., Carlyle, J. (2006). Primary care counsellors' experiences of working with treatment resistant depression: A qualitative pilot study. *Counselling and Psychotherapy Research, 6*(4), 250–257.

McWilliams, N. (2011). *Psychoanalytic diagnosis: Understanding personality structure in the clinical process* (2nd ed.). The Guilford Press.

Najavits, L. M. (2000). Researching therapist emotions and countertransference. *Cognitive and Behavioral Practice, 7,* 322–328.

Paukert, A. L., Pettit, J. W., Amacker, A. (2008). The role of interdependence and perceived similarity in depressed affect contagion. *Behavior Therapy, 39,* 277–285.

Rahn, E., Mahnkopf, A. (1999). *Lehrbuch Psychiatrie für Studium und Beruf.* Verlag.

Roubal, J., Řiháček, T. (2016). Therapists' in-session experiences with depressive clients: A grounded theory. *Psychotherapy Research, 26*(2), 206–219.

Schröder, T. A., Davis, J. D. (2004). Therapists' experience of difficulty in practice. *Psychotherapy Research, 14*(3), 328–345.

Strack, S., Coyne, J. C. (1983). Social confirmation of dysphoria: Shared and private reactions to depression. *Journal of Personality and Social Psychology, 44,* 798–806.

Strauss, A., Corbin, J. M. (1990). *Basics of qualitative research: Grounded theory procedures and techniques.* Sage.

Williams, E. N., Polster, D., Grizzard, M. B., Rockenbaugh, J., & Judge, A. B. (2003). What happens when therapists feel bored or anxious? A qualitative study of distracting self-awareness and therapists' management strategies. *Journal of Contemporary Psychotherapy*, 33(1), 5–18.

Winer, D., Bonner, T., Blaney, P., Murray, E. (1981). Depression and social attraction. *Motivation and Emotion*, 5, 153–166.

Winnicott, D. W. (1949). Hate in the counter-transference. *International Journal of Psychoanalysis*, 30, 69–74.

Wolf, A. W., Goldfried, M. R., Muran, J. C. (2013). Introduction. In Wolf A. W., Goldfried, M. R., Muran, J. C. (Eds.), *Transforming negative reactions to clients: From frustration to compassion*. American Psychological Association, 269–282.

Chapter 2

We Depress Together

"Every five minutes they check their watch and hope that the session is close to being over. They are with a client who is self-absorbed and barely aware of the therapist's presence. They may start to feel incompetent and begin to criticize themselves. They may even begin to regret choosing a profession that forces them to put the needs of others before their own" (Wolf, Goldfried & Muran, 2013, p. 5). The frustration of psychotherapists probably depends on what expectations they have of being with a depressed client. As psychotherapists, we react to the helplessness of depressed clients and can thus easily, and without fully realizing it, find ourselves in the position of a rescuer taking responsibility for the client's recovery.

A client usually comes to therapy because they don't want to live like this anymore, they can't. They want change. And they are terribly afraid of change. Because the dysfunctionality in their life is also the only thing they know. Change is scary because it is unknown. But it is also not possible to continue living like this. Thus, there is desire for change and fear of it. In this contradicting state, they sit before us and immediately delegate to us the power that is directed toward change. "You understand this, that's what you are here for, help me." They project competence onto us and they are left with powerlessness. And if we accept this projection, the original internal contradiction of the client seems to begin to play out between us. The internal struggle is externalized (Zinker, 1977). We, the therapists, thus take hold of the polarity heading toward change, and the client is left with the polarity of the fear of change. We become the competent one who sees that change is necessary. And the client is left with: "Yes, but…"

This decision, in addition to calcifying the client's discontent state and bolstering the therapist's frustration, allows for an important relational dynamic to take place. It is as if the client is saying:

I long for someone to really hear how sick I feel. I hope it's you, therapist. But you seem to think that it can be handled, that it's not so bad. As if you can't hear how sick I feel. Instead you try to change me. You leave me alone in my misery. So it is necessary to go further and show you even more how poorly I am doing.

By trying to apply change, we leave the client in their fear of change. We leave them abandoned and unheard in their suffering.

DOI: 10.4324/9781003500148-3

We can fall into this trap with various clients. Yet it happens particularly easily with depressive clients. Why? After all, we know it all too well. Why do we find ourselves stuck in this trap again and again? Perhaps we are protecting ourselves, keeping ourselves safe from the experiences that depression brings. Our active attitude, our focus on change, can pull us out of sinking into the experiential swamp of depression. Thus, maybe polarization toward the client protects us from becoming depressed ourselves.

Contagious Depression

The phenomenon "contagious depression" (Coyne, 1976a) describes the transfer of the emotional and behavioral manifestations of depression (low mood, gloom, anhedonia, excessive fatigue, pessimism, etc.) from a depressed person to someone else. Only depressive symptoms are transmitted, which is caused by the specific behavior of depressed people. There are several hypotheses explaining the contagiousness of depression, but they do not sufficiently confirm the causal relationship between depression and its "contagiousness" (Kostínková, 2009).

Existing research indicates that the phenomenon of contagious depression is independent of age, education, financial situation, race or health status (Bookwala & Schulz, 1996), and has also been confirmed across different relationships: strangers, roommates, partners and married couples (Benazon & Coyne, 2000). The closer the relationship with the depressed person, the higher the risk of contagious depression (Goodman & Shippy, 2002).

Joiner and Katz (1999) conducted a meta-analysis of studies on the phenomenon of contagious depression in close relationships, in which they conclude that this phenomenon is sufficiently confirmed in research. Although research describing "contagious depression" in a psychotherapeutic relationship has not yet been conducted, we can assume that similar processes to those occurring in other types of relationships occur between a client and a psychotherapist.

What we experience in the presence of a depressed client can subtly undermine the solid ground under our feet. For example, we may feel warmth toward the client. After all, "depressed clients are easy to like" (McWilliams, 2011, p. 248). However, the client is unable to respond to our warmth due to being subdued by depression. Unbeknownst to us, dissatisfaction and disappointment can then accumulate in us, little by little.

A relationship with a depressed client does not resonate. We invest and get nothing back. Frustration builds up within us, but we keep it to ourselves out of consideration for the client. It is as if our body soaks up the frustration. At the same time, it is as if we ourselves succumb to the subdued state of depression and are unable to do anything about it. Similar experiences can gradually engulf us, a feeling of powerlessness can take control over us. We then begin to doubt whether we are even fit for this profession (in the case of novice psychotherapists) or become cynics disappointed by our own lack of effectiveness (in the case of experienced professionals) (Wolf et al., 2013).

This common clinical experience, which is even described in psychiatric text-books, warns us that when working with a depressed client, our mood can deject and we must be careful not to immerse ourselves too much in our own experience (Rahn & Mahnkopf, 1999). Working with depressed clients can not only undermine our professional confidence, but also threaten us personally. Just a conversation with a depressed person causes the other person increased stress (Gurtman, Martin & Hintzman, 1990). Greater risk of depression is evoked, however, when demands are made on the other to help the depressed person (Marks & Hammen, 1982).

Occupational Injuries in Psychotherapy

A psychotherapist's sense of personal endangerment (which comes into play not only when working with depressed clients) is supported by other evidence as well. In his qualitative study of the countertransference experiences of psychotherapists who were themselves psychiatrically hospitalized, Cain (2000) pointed out that these "wounded healers" also experienced varying degrees of identification with their clients. The authors McCann and Pearlman (1990) found transference of symptoms from the client to the psychotherapist in the case of post-traumatic stress disorder. They found that psychotherapists who had not experienced trauma themselves developed long-term changes in cognitive schemas, beliefs, expectations and flash-backs after undergoing psychotherapeutic work with traumatized clients. That is, they developed symptoms typical of post-traumatic stress disorder.

Based on these findings, the authors formulated the concept of "vicarious traumatization," which does not develop on the basis of experiencing a traumatic event, but as a result of its mediation by the client. Psychotherapists have been found to experience symptoms of both post-traumatic stress disorder and burnout: fatigue, loss of compassion, sleep disturbances, intrusive thoughts and images, strong emotional reactions, and also depression (McCann & Pearlman, 1990).

In applying this concept to the case of depression, we might speak of "vicarious depression." Indeed, depressed clients have a significantly stressful effect on their psychotherapists (Deutsch, 1984). They evoke in them feelings of their own depression (Brody & Farber, 1996). Clients with chronic depression are considered by clinicians to be one of the main types of "difficult clients" for their needy, demanding, self-destructive and dependent behavior (Koekkoek, van Meijel & Hutschemaekers, 2006). Specifically, it is the powerlessness and hopelessness of depressed clients that activates reactions of rejection in their psychotherapists (Levenson, 2013).

It seems then, that we are working in a rather dangerous environment where we ourselves are at risk of contagious depression. It is understandable that we try to protect ourselves with our activeness and optimism. In doing so, we take over the client's projection of competence and desire for change. In a therapeutic relationship, we are the ones trying for a change. The client is left with the other polarity: powerlessness. The same one that endangers us.

In this way, the vicious circle of depression in the therapeutic relationship spins on and on, as we will discuss further. In order to avoid this trap, withstand the tension between the two polarities and be able to meet the client in their dichotomous relationship with change – at once desirous and fearful – we need to manage our own experiences. A theoretical framework can help us. It gives meaning to our experience and enables us to process our experiences with a depressed client. It is therefore important for our anchoring in the psychotherapeutic position to understand what happens during depression. To understand what happens with us in the face of another's depression. And to know our role in all this.

Depression in Someone's Story

What sort of depression we see depends on where we look. First, let us look at a person as an individual. We see a person who has fallen into depression, in which both psychosocial and biological factors are involved. Genetic predisposition is largely responsible for the specific vulnerability of a person to depression, making someone more liable to react in a depressive manner to an excessively stressful situation. A depressed person loses self-confidence, will and motivation for contact with others. They are well aware (almost too well) of their condition, but they are not able to mobilize themselves into actively engaging with the surrounding world. They cannot express their needs externally. They turn their frustration from these unmet needs against themselves, tormenting themselves with unfulfillable demands. In this way, they isolate themselves from their environment and cannot draw strength from nourishing contact with others. This lack of strength then further inhibits them from mobilizing themselves and establishing contact with others. They reel in this vicious circle and see no way out. They feel hopeless, which further weakens them and discourages them from reaching out to others.

Now, let us broaden our view and see this person on the path of their life story. From this wider perspective, depressive experiences may not necessarily be an illness. There are situations when a depressive way of interacting with the given environment is advantageous for the organism. We can imagine that each emotional state regulates the interaction between the organism and the environment in a certain way. In this sense, we do not have to think of depressive functioning as a disorder, but as a specific form of creative adjustment, namely depressive adjustment (Roubal, 2007).

Depression's Low Power Mode

Our emotional states are related not only to our given situations at the time, but also to what is forthcoming. One could say that emotions prepare the organism to handle the upcoming situation effectively (Nesse, 2000). Our emotional system thus "switches" our organism into the mode that is advantageous in the moment.

A functional emotional state that outwardly resembles depression can be called a low mood (Nesse, 2000). It is not just a change in mood, but an overall reset of the organism to a "low power mode," during which activity is limited, energy wanes and experiential intensity reduces. These are symptoms identical to those of depression, yet it is not a pathological disorder, but an adaptive mechanism. A sad person conserves their personal resources (Nesse, 2000).

Depressive experiencing also helps us abandon unproductive efforts. This is evident, for example, in the case of a client who comes to us with depressive experiences following an abortion. The depressive experience temporarily slows the woman down. She does not immediately and optimistically try for another pregnancy. Instead, she withdraws from her partner and lacks interest in sex. Her organism is not yet ready for another pregnancy, and depressive adjustment helps to take a break.

In the context of a life story, we can sometimes understand the depressive experience as preparation for what is to come later in life. Therefore, depression often appears in transitional periods of life, for example when stepping into adulthood or old age. It can serve as a certain form of life respite, a time for rearranging priorities and redirecting to the next chapter. In certain life situations, one simply does not have the opportunity to fulfill one's needs, and effective action is not possible. In such cases, we see how the depressive experience economically regulates one's personal investment and limits activity that would be wasted.

The story of Richard is very illustrative in this regard. He was an extremely hard-working, ambitious office worker who persistently rose to higher and higher positions in his company for years. Then his progress stagnated for some time. He continued to work hard for the next promotion. He was very eager for a managerial position. However, in the final round of interviews, he was not selected for the position.

After some time, he came to psychotherapy in a very depressed state: tired, ineffective, without any interest in life around him or in his career. We can understand this as a reaction of his organism in the given situation to not waste energy striving for a leading position that was unattainable at the time. A depressive form of creative adjustment to the situation allowed him to withdraw into sadness and solitude. One could say that he was having a "time-out," during which he had the opportunity to consider his altered life situation in the wider context of his entire life story and to look for alternative strategies.

Moreover, if Richard had persisted in working on getting promoted despite his failed attempt, communicating with him would require a lot of wasted energy from his colleagues in the office. With his depressive adjustment, he saved energy for his entire company. Thus, his creative adjustment was beneficial both for him personally and for those around him at the time.

The Social Function of Depressive Experiencing

Optimism usually helps when dealing with difficult situations. However, there are also situations that only get worse with an optimistic approach. In these cases, it is more advantageous to turn down the effort and demonstrate resignation. For example, when one comes into conflict with a dominant individual and cannot succeed vis-à-vis this individual (Price, 1967). Here we see that the approach is one of "depressive adjustment," which inhibits dangerous and unnecessary action at a time when the organism does not have sufficient internal resources or lacks a feasible life strategy for the given situation.

This kind of depressive adjustment has significance not only for individuals but also for society as a whole. The sociobiological perspective shows the social function of the depressive syndrome as an adaptive mechanism (Nesse, 2000). It is based on ethological theory, according to which aggression is an integral part of the emotional toolbox of animals (Lorenz, 2003). However, in a dense population, aggression can become destructive; therefore, certain mechanisms exist to mitigate its dangerous consequences. One such mechanism is the social stratification of dominance hierarchy (Price, 1967).

Descent in the social hierarchy occurs in the event of injury, illness, old age, or the loss of a loved one. At such times, a person shows symptoms that manifest as depression. It might seem that a sad person is doomed to failure and is not even an asset to the community. Nevertheless, this sad way of relating occurs often and can be traced throughout the history of the human race. Selection pressures have helped keep this way of interacting with the environment throughout evolution as advantageous, as a sad mood provides both protection to the individual and benefit to the community as a whole. When an individual loses interest in their further destiny, they do not fight for it and are thus not injured or killed. Moreover, if they voluntarily relinquish their social position, they also save the community the energy necessary for fighting for each step in the social hierarchy (Price, 1967). Depressive adjustment thus serves in situations of social descent as an adaptation mechanism, whereby a sad mood provides protection for the individual and benefits the entire community.

The emotions that arise during a depressive experience are thus not necessarily symptomatic of a depressive illness. Depressive symptoms do not necessarily signify a pathological problem if we view them as part of a life story. It is especially a person's support system that determines whether a depressive state will serve as a functional adaptation. Or if in fact the person will get stuck in a vicious circle of depression, which no longer helps in adapting to a given situation, but only further weakens their organism. An initially helpful adaptive mechanism of depressive adjustment can develop into a limiting rigid pattern that locks a person into a prison of depressive functioning regardless of their life situation.

Depression in Relationships

We can now broaden our view even further. Instead of focusing on the individual, let us look at relationships. We can see that relationships with the depressed person become organized in a depressive manner. People around the depressed person co-create a depressive relationship arrangement and at the same time are themselves influenced by it. Yes, people co-experience depression: in contact with a depressed person, the conversation stalls, time drags on, and everyone feels weighed down and tired. At the same time, the other people themselves actively contribute to the depression.

Typically, they first try to encourage the depressed person, mobilize them and get them out of the depression: "Come on, it's not that bad. Come on, let's go somewhere. You'll have something else to think about!" But a depressed person at that moment has no capacity to enjoy anything, to be active, to alter their thoughts or their mood. They nevertheless allow themselves to be persuaded and go out into society, function as if a machine, remain closed in on themselves and experience failure once again. This relationship experience further destroys their hope that getting out of their excruciating loneliness could even be possible and causes them to fall further and further into the whirlpool of depression.

Their loved ones are also frustrated by such a failure. They tire of the effort and lose their capacity to further help the depressed person recover. They resign. They need to protect themselves, they start to focus more on their own needs and activities. The depressed person perceives this as another abandonment and once again experiences their own failure. The vicious cycle of depression, this time on an interpersonal level, continues to spin.[1]

The Vicious Cycle of Depression in Relationships

The vicious cycle of depression-reinforcing interactions was explored and described by Coyne (1976a). He attributes the main role in this process to reassurance seeking and rejection by others. People close to a depressed person first respond favorably to their significant need for support and validation with support and compassion. But a depressed person continues to look for support, which evokes feelings of guilt and hostility toward them in the people around them. The other people are ashamed of these experiences, try to suppress them and try to help alleviate the person's depressive symptoms. They attempt to lessen their own feelings of guilt by providing insincere comfort and support to the depressed person. However, at the same time, they indirectly reject the depressed person and avoid them because they find the interaction unpleasant. This contradiction further confirms the depressed person's belief that they are not accepted. They respond by requiring additional support and reassurance, which in turn creates a vicious cycle of interpersonal interactions.

Thus, if we shift the focus from the individual to what happens in the relational "between," we can see that the relationship suffers in depression[2] (Francesetti & Roubal, 2013). In a depressive relationship, there is an existential desire for closeness to the other person. At the same time, there is a strongly experienced loss of hope that it might ever be possible to get close to the other, and thereby get out of the deserted emptiness. This combination of experiences creates deep mental pain, thereby crippling and draining everyone involved in the depressive relationship.

This is also true in a therapeutic situation. As therapists, we cannot position ourselves outside of the relationship with our client. Just like other people in the presence of a depressed person, we also experience and participate in creating a relationship with them. Psychotherapy is not about contact between a healthy professional and a client disturbed by depression. It is us who become "the other" for the client in the moment. We represent the client's general experience with others. We represent all the others whom the client longs to reach and yet who are hopelessly unreachable from the depths of depression.

Thus, relational suffering is actualized in our therapeutic relationship with the client. The unreachability of the other and the loss of hope are also present between us. We as therapists experience them too. Together with the client, we create a vicious cycle of depression, in which our lack of energy prevents us from establishing mutually satisfying and invigorating interactions that would give way to the experience of truly encountering another person.

One could say that the client and the therapist are *depressing together* in the here and now (Roubal, 2007). Both participate in the deformation of relational processes by pulling away from the constantly created bond that connects people to the world and life (Francesetti & Roubal, 2013). Their relationship suffers and they experience the effects within themselves. As we can clearly observe, the client experiences it as symptoms of depression. The therapist experiences fatigue, hopelessness, exhaustion and powerlessness. The therapist reacts by trying to be the savior (of both the other and themselves), thereby further strengthening the vicious interpersonal cycle of depression. Together they sink into the swamp of depression.

We Have No Choice

"Emotional contagiousness" can be explained by the continuous automatic imitation and synchronization of behavioral displays of emotion (Hatfield, Cacioppo & Rapson, 1993) that occur naturally and often unconsciously. Levenson (2013, p. 2014) describes how these "automatic" and "universal" emotional responses also manifest on a physical level, and argues that the therapist largely has no choice whether to control or express them.

Neuroscientific findings suggest that the psychotherapist's brain "immediately pairs" (Thompson, 2001, p. 9) with the client's brain, even before the psychotherapist notices or can consciously influence it. In the therapist's brain, thanks to mirror neurons (Gallese & Goldman, 1998), "a neuronal representation of the other person's mental state is created," which is then used for "internal simulation" (Siegel, 2012, p. 176). This "internal simulation" of the client's mental state leads to the psychotherapist co-experiencing depression with the client. Due to the automatic nature of such a response, the psychotherapist likely cannot avoid it, even if they have previously experienced it and reflected on it in their work.

The Depressive Field Drags Us Down

It appears that psychotherapists cannot avoid their own reactions to depression. Indeed, it would even be detrimental to psychotherapy to skip this initial attunement to the client, as it creates a valuable "gateway to empathy" (Siegel, 2012, p. 165) and opens the "intersubjectivity of consciousness" (Thompson, 2001, p. 15). The therapist's experience in itself thus provides valuable and otherwise unattainable information about the larger whole, which we here call the field.

We can now broaden our view of depression even more and perceive the depressive situation in its entirety (Lewin, 1952), which goes beyond the individuals and their relationship. The whole of a situation is more than just the meeting of two people. The psychotherapeutic situation as a whole is qualitatively different from the sum of its parts. Something new comes into being, which belongs to the given situation and goes beyond the mere sum of the experiences of the client and the experiences of the therapist.

We can imagine the added part as a certain "mycelium" of a depressive situation. It is a meta-phenomenon with its own dynamics, which itself shapes the participants of the given situation. The situation changes from moment to moment and this process has its own dynamics. It is the field's way of organizing itself that transforms both the client and the therapist. They are both a function of the dynamics of the depressed organization of the field. We see them being pulled into the swamp of depression by the field's forces that are beyond their grasp. It is this perspective that we mainly focus on throughout the remainder of this book.

Notes

1 The interpersonal concept of depression differs in each psychotherapeutic approach according to the specifics of the given theory. What they all have in common is the assumption that people suffering from depression and the people close to them have mutually unfulfilling, even stressful relationships with one another, and that these are the key factors in maintaining and worsening depressive episodes (Siegel & Alloy, 1990).

2 Often in this book, I draw ideas or inspiration from texts that Gianni and I wrote together (especially: Francesetti & Roubal, 2013; Francesetti & Roubal, 2020; Roubal & Francesetti, 2022). I tried to source from the parts that I contributed; however, sometimes it is impossible to separate Gianni's contribution from my own, because our texts were created by thinking together and aligning our views. So I would like to thank Gianni Francesetti and express appreciation for his impressive influence on contemporary Gestalt therapy. I further refer the reader to his own texts, e.g. the book specifically about depression *Absence Is the Bridge Between Us* (Francesetti, 2013) or more generally about psychopathology *Neither Inside Nor Outside: Psychopathology and Atmospheres* (Francesetti and Griffero, 2019).

Bibliography

Baume S. (2015). *Spill simmer falter wither*. Tramp Press, p. 42.

Benazon, N. R, Coyne, J. C. (2000). Living with a depressed spouse. *Journal of Family Psychology*, 14, 71–79.

Bookwala, J., Schulz, R. (1996). Spousal similarity in subjective well-being: The cardiovascular health study. *Psychology and Aging,* 11, 582–590.

Brody, E. M., Farber, B. A. (1996). The effects of therapist experience and patient diagnosis on countertransference. *Psychotherapy*, 33(3), 372–380.

Cain, N. R. (2000). Psychotherapists with personal histories of psychiatric hospitalization: Countertransference in wounded healers. *Psychiatric Rehabilitation Journal*, 24(1), 22–28.

Coyne, J. C. (1976a). Depression and the response of others. *Journal of Abnormal Psychology*, 85, 186–193.

Coyne, J. C. (1976b). Toward an interactional description of depression. *Psychiatry*, 39, 28–40.

Deutsch, C. J. (1984). Self-reported sources of stress among psychotherapists. *Professional Psychology: Research and Practice*, 15(6), 833–845.

Francesetti, G. (2015). *Absence is the bridge between us*. Intituto di Gestalt HCC.

Francesetti, G., Griffero, T. (2019). *Neither inside nor outside: Psychopathology and atmospheres*. Cambridge Scholars Publishing.

Francesetti, G., Roubal, J. (2013) Gestalt therapy approach to depressive experiences. In Francesetti, G., Gecele, M., Roubal, J. (Eds.), *Gestalt therapy in clinical practice: From psychopathology to the aesthetics of contact*. Franco Angeli, 433–494.

Francesetti, G., Roubal, J. (2020). Field theory in contemporary Gestalt therapy, Part 1: Modulating the therapist's presence in clinical practice. *Gestalt Review*, 24(2), 113–136.

Gallese, V., Goldman, A. (1998). Mirror neurons and the simulation theory of mind-reading. *Trends in Cognitive Sciences*, 2, 493–501.

Goodman, C. R., Shippy, R. A. (2002). Is it contagious? Affect similarity among spouses. *Aging and Mental Health*, 6, 266–274.

Gurtman, M. B., Martin, K. M., Hintzman, N. M. (1990). Interpersonal reactions to displays of depression and anxiety. *Journal of Social and Clinical Psychology*, 9, 256–267.

Hatfield, E., Cacioppo, J. L., Rapson, R. L. (1993). Emotional contagion. *Current Directions in Psychological Sciences*, 2, 96–99.

Joiner, T. E., Katz, J. (1999). Contagion of depressive symptoms and mood: Meta-analytic review and explanations from cognitive, behavioral, and interpersonal viewpoints. *Clinical Psychology and Science Practice*, 6, 149–164.

Koekkoek, B., van Meijel, B., Hutschemaekers, G. (2006). "Difficult patients" in mental health care: A review. *Psychiatric Services*, 57(6), 795–802.

Kostínková, J. (2009). *Zkušenost ženy v partnerství s mužem nemocným depresí [Experiences of a woman in partnership with a depressed man].* MU FSS, Katedra psychologie.

Levenson, H. (2013). Time-limited dynamic psychotherapy: Working with reactions to chronically depressed clients. In Wolf, A. W., Goldfried, M. R., Muran, J. C (Eds.), *Transforming negative reactions to clients: From frustration to compassion.* American Psychological Association, 191–219.

Lewin, K. (1952). *Field theory in social science: Selected theoretical papers.* Harper and Brothers.

Lorenz, K. (2003). *Takzvané zlo [orig.: Das sogenannte Böse, 1963].* Academia.

Marks, T., Hammen, C. L. (1982). Interpersonal mood induction: Situational and individual determinants. *Motivation and Emotion*, 6, 387–399.

McCann, I. L., Pearlman, L. A. (1990). Vicarious traumatization: A framework for understanding the psychological effects of working with victims. *Journal of Traumatic Stress*, 3(1), 131–149.

McWilliams, N. (2011). *Psychoanalytic diagnosis: Understanding personality structure in the clinical process* (2nd ed.). The Guilford Press.

Nesse, R. M. (2000). Is depression an adaptation? *Archives of General Psychiatry*, 57, 14–20.

Price, J. (1967). The dominance hierarchy and the evolution of mental illness. *Lancet*, II(7502), 243–246.

Rahn, E., Mahnkopf, A. (1999). *Lehrbuch Psychiatrie für Studium und Beruf.* Verlag.

Roubal, J. (2007). Depression – a Gestalt theoretical perspective. *British Gestalt Journal*, 16(1), 35–43.

Roubal, J., Francesetti, G. (2022). Field theory in contemporary Gestalt therapy, Part 2: Paradoxical theory of change reconsidered. *Gestalt Review*, 26(1), 1–33.

Siegel, D. J. (2012). *The developing mind: How the relationships and the brain interact to shape who we are* (2nd ed.). The Guilford Press.

Siegel, J., Alloy, L. B. (1990). Interpersonal perceptions and consequences of depressive-significant other relationships: A naturalistic study of college roommates. *Journal of Abnormal Psychology*, 99, 361–373.

Thompson, E. (2001). Empathy and consciousness. *Journal of Consciousness Studies*, 8(5–7), 1–32.

Wolf, A. W., Goldfried, M. R., Muran, J. C. (2013). Introduction. In Wolf, A. W., Goldfried, M. R., Muran, J. C. (Eds.), *Transforming negative reactions to clients: From frustration to compassion.* American Psychological Association, 269–282.

Zinker, J. (1977). *Creative process in Gestalt therapy.* Brunner-Mazel.

Chapter 3

Why Do We Do It?

Again and again I am with someone in depression. "Why am I even doing this?" goes through my head when they leave. Psychotherapy may seem like a good enough choice for a comfortable and safe profession. We therapists sit inside where it's warm, where the rain can't get us, we listen and talk, we drink tea – and we earn a pretty decent living by doing so. Good, right? Especially since it gets easier with age, as grey hair and wrinkles do a lot of work for us. Moreover, it is a profession that by its very nature encourages us to grow.

However, this impression of coziness and safety is rather deceptive. It is a dangerous profession with a high risk of occupational injuries, sometimes with permanent consequences. Specifically, when working with depression, psychotherapists can be understood as high risk workers who are themselves at risk of depression, which is also one of the most common manifestations of a professional crisis for psychotherapists (Gilroy et al., 2002).

The fact that the danger of our work cannot be seen increases the risk even more. It is like there is a battle going on in our office. Clients bring extremely hurtful experiences, harrowing emotions, rage, frustration and their own and others' anger. In other words, all that has long been accumulating in them and can now be released. And so while we sit in our chair and drink tea, grenades of emotions fly around our heads and explode in our cozy study. Unspoken and unfelt emotions simmer in the corners. Fear and terror erupt, murderous aggression hisses at the whole world, and then the air is filled with resentment over wasted years of life.

We sit there, smile and mostly have no notion of job security. We don't protect ourselves, we don't have work attire and tools. Quite the opposite. We are trained to expose ourselves to murderous bullets. To open up with empathy. We run around the battlefield naked. And we even encourage it all: *yes, hit me, tell me more about it.*

To make matters worse: we don't even really have control over it. As neuroscience informs us, the client's brain pairs with our own – they connect to one another. We could say that the more damaged brain is being repaired by the healthier one.[1] Most likely, the client's brain is repairing itself via ours, synchronizing and harmonizing with it. Good for them. But what is happening to our brain?

Why didn't anyone warn us that in psychotherapy the therapist's health is at risk? Only after years of work-related injuries draining us of so much strength are we

DOI: 10.4324/9781003500148-4

forced to take notice. Until then, we probably operate mainly on beginner's enthusiasm and the helping profession's idealism. Then we realize that we have to start protecting ourselves. That we probably need to shield ourselves against harmful bullets.

Yet, wouldn't we then lose the key element needed for our work? Would we not lose sensitivity to the suffering of others? Perhaps armor would only escalate the war. Could it not be done differently? Might it be possible to dance between the bullets? Perhaps, paradoxically, our years of trained sensitivity would help us. We would sense a dangerous emotional bullet flying toward us and we would avoid it with an aikido move. This approach requires a somewhat different training from what we had and have. How do you dance in a depressive field? How do you work with a client in such a flexible, dancing way?

Psychotherapeutic Change

We can have a sitting with our client in various ways. Just like our body on a chair, we can adjust our mind. It depends on how we approach what happens in psychotherapy. We can set our position by how we give meaning to what we do. How we explain to ourselves why clients actually come to us, what our psychotherapy work is about and what our role is.

Perhaps it would be possible to say on a very general level that clients come to us for psychotherapy because they desire change. Such change can take on different forms from person to person, but what is important for us is that clients are not able to achieve this change on their own. Their current life situation brings them troubles of various kinds, and they hope that psychotherapy will improve their lives. We, psychotherapists, take clients in for therapy and start working with them. By doing so, we implicitly commit ourselves to helping them achieve the desired change. As psychotherapists, we therefore take some part of responsibility for the change that happens in psychotherapy.

However, the situation is far from simple. Clients may desire to change something that cannot be achieved in therapy (to get their wife to come back to them; to get rid of their anxiety, etc.). Often, they only fully realize what they want to change during the therapy session. At the same time, therapists likewise cannot plan in advance what form the therapeutic change will take and how it will develop. Therefore, as we continuously adapt our work to the changing psychotherapeutic process, our commitment, which we take on as therapists by accepting clients into therapy, assumes an indefinite form. We agree to help the clients with change, but neither they nor we have any clear idea of it in advance.

What is more, we are present in the meeting with the client not only as professionals helping with the process of change. We are also present as perceptive human beings, who are experientially exposed to extremely powerful situations in the clinical setting. Encountering psychopathology deforms us experientially: a depressive situation pulls us down, a panic situation opens up the ground under our feet, a psychotic situation blurs the contours of our world, an obsessive-compulsive situation constricts us, a traumatic situation stuns us. In the situation here and now, together with the client, we become part of the dynamics of the depressive, psychotic, panic, obsessive compulsive, traumatic or other psychopathological field. Although of course it is true that in addition to the aforementioned common features, the suffering of each client also has an individual nature. So each clinical situation uniquely troubles us therapists.

We experience all this voluntarily and for good reason. We choose not to protect ourselves with our knowledge, diagnostic skills, professional experience or authority. We do not wear a white coat to therapy. We open up in interpersonal contact, which allows us to enter into the suffering of another and be present in the suffering actualized in the here and now. In order to reach the client as a human being, not just a set of symptoms, it seems inevitable that we "risk ourselves" in this way (Rogers, in Anderson, 1997, p. 85).

At the same time, in order to prevent the turbulence of the clinical situation from experientially rattling us too much, it is good to have something firm to hold on to. Being alone in a meeting with a client is risky. We need a strong supporting third party in the therapeutic relationship (Francesetti, Gecele & Roubal, 2013). For this role, we can employ our experience, knowledge and authority. However, we do not use them as a shield protecting us from the personal threat posed to us by a clinical situation. Rather, we cling to them like to the rails of a ship, allowing us to flow with the movement of the situation and simultaneously take care of our own safety. The process of change often unfolds in an unexpected and unpredictable direction, and we therefore need our own meaningful *theory of change*, with the help of which we are able to grasp the process of change.

A tremendous number of processes take place on many levels in a psychotherapeutic meeting. In addition to the two people physically present, we can imagine that the ancestors of both the client and the therapist are also present through the relationship patterns passed down over generations. It is as if they, too, join us in the meeting – our grandmothers and grandfathers mingle with the client. Various other influences come implicitly into play as well, such as the social atmosphere, cultural and spiritual traditions, but also autonomous physical stimuli, such as mutual reactions to smell sensations between the client and the therapist. More and more influences come into being at each moment and participate in the therapy process.

Clearly, a huge number of factors are at play. That is why change in psychotherapy is so complex, and we will probably never fully understand all that changes. It is similar to how our hearing apparatus can only pick up sounds of a certain wavelength. There are far more sounds than we register, we just do not have the opportunity to hear them directly. Of all the various processes involved in the therapeutic situation, we are able to notice only some. All of them though, including the inaudible ones, resonate and contribute to the resulting form of therapeutic change. What's more, therapeutic change interacts with change resulting from factors outside of therapy. Therapeutic change also shifts over time, with some changes only manifesting months or years after therapy.

It seems evident that it is not within our ability to fully grasp and clearly name therapeutic change. The outcome of psychotherapy will probably always remain highly uncertain. But we can learn to understand the processes that take place in psychotherapy and explain the therapeutic change. We can learn to enter these processes in different ways and participate in shaping this change.

How we enter into the process of change as psychotherapists depends on how we understand it – in other words, how we explain what happens in psychotherapy. That depends on our perspective, on the vantage point from where we observe the change process. Our perspective is then fundamentally influenced by the concept of psychopathology and psychotherapy, which is shared in professional circles and which derives from the generally shared thinking patterns of the society of our time (paradigms).

Development of Paradigms

Evans (2007) connects the development of psychotherapy with three paradigms in the history of the West: classical, modern and postmodern. *"God is; therefore I am"* could be paraphrased as a *classical paradigm* that includes the Platonic conception of reality and is based on the idea of transcendence in the Jewish and Christian traditions. Descartes' *"I think, therefore I am"* describes the *modern paradigm* since the Enlightenment and represents a shift from theo-centric to rational-centric thinking. The twenty-first century then relativizes what we know, how we know and what we think we know (Evans, 2007), "demystifying the grand narrative of modernism" (Gergen, 1992, p. 28). This *postmodern paradigm* emphasizes the co-creation of relationships, and therefore views the psychotherapeutic relationship as an interactive process in which both parties influence one another: *"You are, therefore I am"* (Evans, 2007).

The concept of paradigm shifts will help us distinguish between different conceptions of the process of change in psychotherapy: How does change happen and who makes it happen? In the modern paradigm, currently prevailing in the Western healthcare system and in its associated psychotherapy, change is brought by an expert who helps the client repair a disorder.

Before that, in the era of the classical paradigm, psychotherapy did not exist as a separate field, but similar processes of change took place in other, mainly spiritual contexts. Change was brought about by the action of an external force, and the expert was competent to ask this force for help. In the postmodern paradigm, which increasingly influences contemporary psychotherapy, we view change as co-created by therapist and client.

We are currently perhaps witnessing the hatching of another, fresh paradigm that follows on from those aforementioned. Conceptually, it refers to *field theory*. Field theory itself is not new. It is mainly based on the work of Kurt Lewin (1952) and resonates with the epistemology of various psychotherapeutic approaches, not only Gestalt therapy, but also, for example, contemporary psychoanalysis (Ogden, 2003; Katz, 2016; Ferro & Civitarese, 2016).

From its very inception, Gestalt therapy built its conceptual foundation on field theory, which thus informs the theory and practice of the Gestalt approach (Perls, Hefferline & Goodman, 1951). Field theory functions in Gestalt therapy as the "cognitive glue" that holds the Gestalt therapy system together (Yontef, 1993). It is currently being newly developed with regard to ongoing changes in the social, cultural and scientific context. It seems that field theory has the potential to be a shared concept in contemporary psychotherapy and thus contribute to the shift from the pre-paradigmatic stage to the establishment of a new paradigm where the professional community shares a basic theoretical background (Evans, 2007).

Simply put, we could say that field theory describes the dynamics of a whole that is greater than the sum of its parts. It tries not to limit our perception of reality by separating the organism from the environment, the client from the therapist. Thanks to this, it can then focus on events that transcend such separations. Field theory offers a perspective from which we see how all aspects of a given situation are being organized and constantly rearranged. It then attempts to describe the regularities of the processes by which the field is organized. For the practice of a Gestalt therapist, this means a radical focus on process. On how things happen. And freeing ourselves from trying to explain why they happen. The therapist observes experiential shifts in the situation here and now with the client, but does not attribute them to the individual participants of the situation. Instead, they view them from the perspective of the larger whole, watching moment by moment as the process of field organization unfolds.[2]

In field theory, change is not made by a person, but is a process with its own dynamics that transcends the people involved in the change process. Change happens and this process "uses" the people involved to make itself happen (Roubal, 2019). From this point of view, not only the modern but also the postmodern concept of dialogic co-creation of change still seems too anthropocentric. Perhaps even uncritically omnipotent: you and I make a difference together. How can we be so sure?

The field theory paradigm goes further and humbly acknowledges that change can happen in ways we do not intend or control. It can happen in ways that we sometimes do not understand and that neither side may even notice. Both client and therapist participate in change in a complex, constantly varying manner. At the same time, they themselves are functions of this change as processes that are shaped by the flow of the situation as a whole. The field theory perspective offers contemporary psychotherapy an emphasis on humility toward the healing process that transcends the persons involved.[3]

How to paraphrase the field theory paradigm? Maybe something along the lines of: *"You and I are shaped by our meeting."* It may remind us of the classic paradigm *"God is, therefore I am."* Indeed, both of these paradigms are based on the experience that change is shaped by a power that transcends humans. However, from the perspective of field theory, this force is freed from the religious ideas that prescribe how we should perceive it. Its perception is based purely on the experience of participation in the flow of the given present situation, on the holistically experienced flow of co-existence. "We perceive no You, yet we feel ourselves addressed and we respond… with our being" (Buber, 1937, p. 6).

Notes

1 "The mirror properties in our brains enable us to imagine empathically what is going on inside another person. Internal simulation – the process of absorbing and resonating with others' internal states – is thought to be the first stage of compassion, or "feeling with" other persons" (Siegel, 2012, pp. 165–166). "In trying to understand and accept the perspective of a suffering person, therapists suffer themselves, and the result of such constant attunement can be "compassion fatigue" (Figley, 2002).
2 Field theory is developed in Gestalt therapy in partially different ways (Staemmler, 2006). The original concept of the organism-environment field (Perls, Hefferline, & Goodman, 1951) following the concept of Kurt Lewin (1952) is further developed in the specific concept of the situation (Robine, 2011). Alongside this, the holistic concept of Jan Smuts (1926) develops, and in order to understand field processes, this concept assumes that there is a certain "field energy in the space between" (Parlett, 2005, p. 60). This book also leans toward this concept. For more details, I refer to two related articles on the current conception of field theory in Gestalt therapy (Francesetti & Roubal, 2020; Roubal & Francesetti, 2022).
3 The growing interest in altered states of consciousness associated with the use of psychedelics in psychotherapy can also be understood as a report of a newly emerging paradigm. Humility in the face of forces beyond one's intentions is also essential for working with these states.

Bibliography

Anderson, H. (1997). *Conversation, language, and possibilities: A postmodern approach to therapy*. Basic Books.

Buber, M. (1937). *I and thou*. T. and T. Clark.

Evans, K. (2007). Living in the 21st century: A gestalt therapist's search for a new paradigm. *Gestalt Review*, 11(3), 190–203.

Ferro, A., Civitarese, G. (2016). Psychoanalysis and the analytic field. In Elliott, A., Prager, J. (Eds.), *The Routledge handbook of psychoanalysis in the social sciences and humanities*. Routledge.

Figley, C. R. (2002). Compassion fatigue: Psychotherapists' chronic lack of self care. *Journal of Clinical Psychology*, 58(11), 1433–1441.

Francesetti, G., Roubal, J. (2020). Field theory in contemporary Gestalt therapy, Part 1: Modulating the therapist's presence in clinical practice. *Gestalt Review*, 24(2), 113–136.

Francesetti, G., Gecele, M., & Roubal, J. (2013). Gestalt therapy approach to psychopathology. In Francesetti, G., Gecele, M., & Roubal, J. (Eds.), *Gestalt therapy in clinical practice: From psychopathology to the aesthetics of contact*. FrancoAngeli, 59–76.

Gergen, K. J. (1992). Towards a postmodern psychology. In Kvale, S. (Ed.), *Psychology and postmodernism: Inquiries in social construction*. Sage.

Gilroy, P. J., Murra, J., & Carroll, L. (2002). A preliminary survey of counselling psychologists' personal experiences with depression and treatment. *Professional Psychology: Research & Practice*, 33(4), 402–407.

Katz, M. S. (2016). *Contemporary psychoanalytic field theory: Stories, dreams, and metaphor*. Routledge.

Lewin, K. (1952). *A dynamic theory of personality: Selected papers*. McGraw-Hill.

Ogden, T. H. (2003). What's true and whose idea was it? *The International Journal of Psychoanalysis*, 84(3), 593–606.

Parlett, M. (2005). Contemporary Gestalt therapy: Field theory. In Woldt, A. L., Toman, M. (Ed.), *Gestalt therapy: History, theory, and practice*. Sage Publications, 41–64.

Perls, F., Hefferline, R. F., Goodman, P. (1951). *Gestalt therapy: Excitement and growth in the human personality*. Julian Press.

Robine, J. M. (2011). *On the occasion of an other.* Gestalt Journal Press.

Rosa, J. G. (1956*). Noites do Sertão.* Global. [English translation by M. Beránková for the purposes of this book.]

Roubal, J. (2019). Theory of change. In Francesetti, G., Vázquez Bandín, C., Reed, E. (Eds.), *Obsessive-compulsive experiences: A Gestalt therapy.* Los Libros del CTP, 9–20.

Roubal, J., Francesetti, G. (2022). Field theory in contemporary Gestalt therapy, Part 2: Paradoxical theory of change reconsidered. *Gestalt Review*, 26(1), 1–33.

Siegel, D. J. (2012). *The developing mind: How the relationships and the brain interact to shape who we are* (2nd ed.). The Guilford Press.

Smuts, C. J. (1926). *Holism and evolution.* Macmillan; Gestalt Journal Press, 2013.

Staemmler, F.-M. (2006). A Babylonian confusion? On the uses and meanings of the term "field." *British Gestalt Journal*, 15(2), 64–83.

Yontef, G. (1993). *Awareness, dialogue and process: Essays on Gestalt therapy.* Gestalt Journal Press.

Chapter 4

Therapists in the Depressive Swamp

Ugh, I've really had enough today, I can't take it much longer. This session with Daniel should hopefully be over soon. I discreetly glance at the clock and am horrified that only ten minutes have passed since the start of the session! It's like I'm in another world where time crawls ominously slowly. Like I'm wading through deep mud, sinking deeper and deeper with each step. I can't imagine how I'll survive until the end of the session... if the end ever comes. I can't think of any therapeutic interventions. What could I do? And if I do think of something, I don't believe that it could help the client who is sitting across from me. Hopelessness, powerlessness. My creativity has left me and I'm beginning to doubt that what I do can be of use to anyone at all. Certainly not to this client, that's quite clear. And somehow psychotherapy in general makes no sense... It's as if something is draining my energy. I feel low, I am struggling with sleepiness, I am fatigued and sense a heaviness in my whole body...

I'm simply sinking into the swamp of depression together with the client, and the more I try to jump out, the deeper I sink. So for a start, let me try not to get out quickly. Second, let me get a good look around, see what is actually going on, where am I? Yes, I am stuck in a deep swamp and the gooey mud of depression is pulling me in. And I am experiencing this because I chose to work as a psychotherapist with this client. What is happening to me is related to the client's depression and my work. I am experiencing firsthand what it's like for them to be stuck in depression. But I get a taste of it for fifty minutes (however endless those minutes may seem) while they are always stuck in it. Ugh!

While I've been engrossed in these thoughts, time has jumped forward a bit and at least I didn't sink deeper into the swamp. I even look at the client with interest: How do they survive this? How does one manage to move through the mud, day after day, week after week, month after month? And how is it possible that in ten minutes of contact with them, I find myself in the same mud? What was going on within me, what was going on between us? This curiosity seems to revive me somewhat. I still don't know what to do with the client, but at least the terrible heaviness and sleepiness has waned a bit.

DOI: 10.4324/9781003500148-5

Let us now try to examine this psychotherapist's experience of a specific clinical situation in more detail. What is going on with the therapist? The research project "The Experience of Therapists during Psychotherapy Sessions with Depressed Clients," which was described in the first chapter, suggests a general pattern. A pattern that repeats itself and allows us to understand the specific experience of the therapist in a certain situation.

The therapists in the research described their experience in relation to a client's depressive experience as either similar or opposite. They used the metaphor of "experiential distance" between therapist and client. They moved closer to the client or away from them. In the presence of a depressed client, therapists felt that their experience was being "diverted" without their own intention and control. Sometimes they felt "drawn into" the depressive co-experience, at other times they felt "repelled" from it. They were often unaware of this during the actual therapy sessions and discovered it only during the research interview. It was thus possible to conclude that these experiential reactions in the therapeutic situation were largely automatic and unconscious at the given moment.

When therapists experienced being "drawn into" a depressive experience, they noted that their experience was transformed and different from how they usually perceive themselves:

> *I couldn't detach myself from the contact with [the client]. And I recognized in myself, that I had reached some level that is not my own... The level of my mood (...) [which goes] down, when I am there with the client.*[1]

We see that the experiences of the therapists begin to resemble the experiences of their depressed client: *"I feel that they are pulling me down, into some kind of despair... into some kind of black hole."* Therapists began to feel hopeless and incompetent, and they blamed themselves for failing. Thus, they exhibited symptoms present in depression, which shows how close their experience was to the depressive experience of their clients. The experiential distance between them and the client grew smaller.

Yet the therapists also observed the opposite tendency, when they felt repelled from their client. They began to worry about themselves. *"Don't drown in it with them! (...) Don't drown (...) in that issue, in that experience, in that hopelessness."* They felt a tendency to escape, to end the contact with the client. They began to feel dissatisfaction, mistrust, frustration and anger toward the client: *"It actually provokes such a defensive reaction in me, it irritates me. How did it get into me!?"*

We can observe how therapists are constantly drawn into identifying with the experience of depressed clients. At the same time, we see how they are repelled and take an experiential position of polarity toward the client. This process of the therapist's *experiential oscillation* between two poles gradually develops over the course of the therapy session. From the research, it was possible to distinguish individual phases of this trajectory and their typical sequence as depicted in

to depressive experience ← **THERAPIST'S EXPERIENCE** → from depressive experience

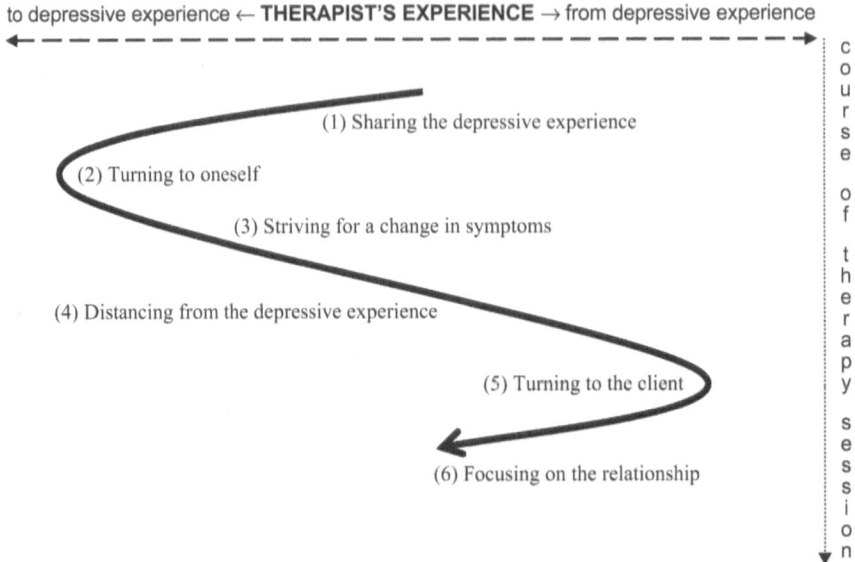

Figure 4.1 Depression Co-Experiencing Trajectory model (Roubal & Řiháček, 2016)

the general Depression Co-Experiencing Trajectory model (see Figure 4.1). This general sequence of phases occurred one or more times during a single session.

Stage 1: Sharing the Depressive Experience

At the beginning of psychotherapy sessions, the therapist's experience begins to re-semble that of their depressed clients. Therapists experience self-doubt, self-blame, feelings of failure, powerlessness, hopelessness, as well as a general muted feeling and fatigue. In other words, they actually experience symptoms of depression in themselves, as if they were falling into depression together with their clients:

> *"I am aware of the nothingness, the emptiness, the meaninglessness."*
> *"Powerlessness. I can't help him."*
> *"I have no idea what to do about it."*

Therapists lose their distance from their clients' experiences, lack a detached view and a broader perspective, and feel dragged down into depression toward their cli-ents: *"Somehow I get into it. Down. And I say to myself: it's terribly hopeless. No wonder there's no way out of it."* They also experience sadness, anxiety, emptiness, fear for their clients and fear of their own failure. They perceive a loss of the ability to think clearly and concentrate: *"I couldn't even really think clearly."* On a physi-cal level, they experience stiffness, heaviness, weakness, exhaustion and fatigue: *"When I sit there with him, I feel terrible fatigue. (...) I feel like I can't even raise my hand anymore."*

Therapists especially experience hopelessness, that *"nothing has meaning and nothing works,"* and a loss of meaning, both of which they share with clients:

> *"I feel it's completely hopeless. That it's all messed up, that nothing has meaning."*

> *"I myself actually become part of that loss of meaning. I feel that I myself am losing my meaning, after what happens with us there."*

Stage 2: Turning to Oneself

Therapists now get so close to their clients that they stop perceiving themselves and their experience begins to merge with the clients' depressive experience. They realize that it is beginning to endanger them personally: *"The client is dragging me down, it's destroying me."* The co-experiencing of depression escalates until it exceeds the capacity of the therapists. They reach a turning point when they stop tuning in experientially to the clients. Instead, they focus on themselves and instinctively begin to protect themselves: *"Protect myself, yeah. I think the kind of negativity that she has toward herself... I am concerned for myself, if I let that get to me."*

One therapist described how a shared depressive experience distorted his perception of himself. He "emotionally approached" so close to the depressed client that he stopped seeing himself as an expert, someone with the capacity to help.

> *As I get closer to him in those emotions, closer to the client, [there is] a limit where I [say in my mind to the client:] 'You should go see a psychologist, man.' Before I realize that he is actually there [at the psychologist]! (...) I forget that I am there as the psychologist. Because I realize how hard it is for me when he describes [his troubles] to me. And I think that's because of the closeness (...) [And then it helps me] to realize that it's me.*

This *"Returning to oneself"* represented a moment of intense self-awareness for the therapist.

> *I try to straighten up, for example... To be aware of my breath, to simply breathe more... To be in contact with what I am through the body, so that it doesn't sweep me away.*

Stage 3: Striving for a Change in Symptoms

At this point, the experiences of the therapists begin to diverge from the experiences of their depressed clients. Therapists stop sharing the experience with their clients on a personal level and take a more detached, safer position as experts. From this position, they then focus on clients' symptoms of depression. They thereby externalize and depersonalize the depressive experience. This allows them to stop their further descent into co-experiencing depression and gain experiential distance. They try for effective treatment of depression and take responsibility for changing the client's condition. They choose a more directive approach, give their clients practical advice and try to help them solve their problems: *"It leads me to look for a solution."*

Interventions by which therapists try to change the symptoms of depression also serve the therapists themselves as a way of managing their own experience. Above all, as a way to escape the overwhelming feeling of powerlessness:

> *The powerlessness was probably the worst (...) I gave the usual talks [to the client], like: We have to ride it out, you have to wait a while for the drugs to take effect. So, the role of the expert (...). I was doing it for the client and at the same time for myself.*

The depressed client's experience is generally characterized by low mood, fatigue, apathy and hopelessness. Therapists manage their own experience in the presence of such a client by retuning to contrasting experiences in the moment. They actively resist falling into passivity and powerlessness. *"For me, that (...) pumping potential automatically jumps in there. In other words, the more down the person is, the more fiercely I mobilize myself."* Therapists try to give the client optimism, change the attitude the client has toward themselves and the world around them, turn them away from a depressive experience and focus on pleasant and positive things, appreciating the client's qualities.

> *The person mobilizes me. I suddenly become very active, I start inventing, I start having a lot of ideas, I start tending to them, I take care of them. I know it's a bit of a trap that I'm falling into. That it's easier for me than staying with them.*

Therapists then sometimes realize that their intervention, to a large extent, is serving themselves in managing their own experience:

> *That I feel, for example, the weight (...) and at the same time I tell him how important it is for me that... that he allows himself to [bring his own difficult experience into therapy]... I try to [show] the connection with the fact that actually just his coming here has meaning. Like, he's doing something. And many times I have realized that at the moment I was doing it more for myself.*

Stage 4: Distancing from the Depressive Experience

As a therapy session progresses, the therapist's experience develops based on the realization that their efforts to change the client's depressive symptoms are not successful. Their encouragement, activity and optimism do not lead to change; the therapist does not see satisfactory results of their efforts. The client does not change according to their expectations, is still depressed and remains immersed in experiences of emptiness, resignation and hopelessness.

Therapists feel that they are *"pushing their way someplace that is closed,"* that the situation is *"stuck in one place,"* or that the client is

> *stuck... in the same recurring themes and the same repetitive sentences, that nothing has meaning anyway, and that in fact, she will never get rid of it [the depression] anyway, and that the world is kind of bleak and...*

Therapists are impatient and frustrated, they implicitly blame the client for their own failures, they feel angry: *"I'm just so angry. I'm downright pissed off. (...) That immobility, that inertness [annoys me]. [It's like] screaming into a black hole."*

Therapists now distance themselves from the client to the point where they no longer see the client as a person. They see only a bearer of symptoms that do not want to change according to the therapist's expectations:

> *"I feel... that [I would want to say to a client:] 'If you just wanted it a little bit, tried a little bit harder, you could do it!' So, that's what it does to me."*

> *"I ask her [after some time]: 'And how do you feel now?' And she says: 'Even worse.' I consider that my own failure as well. That's also why I'm angry. That I failed to help her."*

> *"I'm actually (...) angry. (...) With him, I feel like kicking him!"*

The therapists demarcate themselves vis-à-vis the client: *"I thought to myself: 'My God, I never want to end up like this.'"* Their experience seems incomprehensible to the therapist or they downplay it:

> *"It seems unreal that something like this [such a depressive state] could exist. It's just an absolutely unbelievable thing for me."*

> *"I balanced it with humor... In those tragic moments I look for something like a tragicomedy (...) It's hard for me to take it seriously."*

Therapists feel like running away from contact with their clients: *"I had the feeling that maybe it would be reasonable to end it [therapy]."* They want to send the depressed clients to other specialists and thus avoid further contact with them.

Stage 5: Turning to the Client

Therapists are now so experientially distant from the depressed client that they cease to be empathetic. They are protecting themselves so much from experiencing depression with the client that they temporarily abandon their helping position:

> *Powerlessness, anger. Feeling like it's pointless. It occurs to me that it would probably be good if he committed the suicide that he keeps talking about... That thought comes to mind. And that stops me! That's exactly the stop sign that throws me back again... [I feel at that moment] such horror and shame.*

Therapists have now reached another turning point. They admit that their efforts to rid the client of depressive symptoms were not successful. They are exhausted and also frustrated because their efforts to cause a change in the client's depression seem futile. They stop aiming for change and come to terms with the current limited possibilities of the client and the entire therapeutic situation. They accept the reality of the client's current condition and begin to change their therapeutic approach:

> *I realize (...) that it is my haste or precipitance or heaviness, that I want it quickly [to change]... So [I start doing it differently and] I'm still there [with him] (...) and I'm more silent. (...) Tune in to his pace. Something like that.*

Therapists abandon the role of the expert who brings about change and simply remain in the presence of the other: *"I can sit with her, but I can't help her."* They stop experientially distancing themselves from the client. They become intensely aware of the presence of the client as a person with whom they are meeting in the now. However, it is not easy, because they experience an internal tension between the natural tendency to protect themselves from a depressive co-experience and their professional responsibility.

Stage 6: Focusing on the Relationship

Now the experiences of the therapists begin to approach the experiences of the depressed clients again. Therapists focus on the relationship instead of the symptoms: *"I'm going to join her. Nothing will improve, we will not reach a solution, we will not reach anything [new], but some contact may occur. I am with her, (...) [there is] some sort of relationship."*

This is not only a change in the therapeutic approach toward the client, but also in the way in which therapists manage their own experiences:

> *Well, I feel that it helps me... when those moments of deeper contact occur. Because I start to perceive it as at least a little meaningful and somehow through it I can like the other person even with all that. It helps that there is not only that darkness, but also, something alive. Something really alive. [It helps me] that there is not only death there (...) [but also] that there's life there... That when I got close to her, I felt not only her depression, but also her as a being.*

Therapists newly define their role in the given situation, allowing them to begin to get closer to the client in an experiential way again: *"That I stop trying to get him moving, but rather join him."* Ceding efforts for a change of symptoms and focusing on the relationship makes work for therapists meaningful again. It brings them relief and allows them to stay with the client:

> *It was a relief... It was quite a relief actually to feel that it [improving depression] was not just some duty. (...) That actually for her the meeting [in itself] (...) has some kind of positive benefit. (...) So that actually helped me quite a bit.*

Therapists experience ambivalence at this stage. On the one hand, they experience relief when they have left an unproductive effort, but at the same time they persist in sharing the unpleasant experience with the client:

It was like finding solid ground. Landing. You stop squirming in some activity, but you just take a seat. So you sit, [but] the wall is impenetrable. On the one hand, it's a relief from the activity, but on the other, you're just sitting there in something bad.

Conclusion of Research Results

The moment of the experiential turn to the client (stage 5) represents a crucial moment in the psychotherapy of depression, which we will discuss in detail later. It is at this very moment that therapists, thanks to their professional responsibility, do not leave the client, but stay with them, even if their efforts to help them are not successful. By remaining with the client at this point, therapists break the interpersonal vicious cycle of depression. They behave differently than how the client experiences the behavior of their loved ones.

We could say that they behave unnaturally, senselessly and even madly: they stay in a situation that is uncomfortable or even dangerous for them. Empty-handed, they turn back to the client. They even go to meet the client, experientially approaching them again (stage 6), but this time in a different way. They voluntarily expose themselves to depression while giving up trying to change it. Thanks to this, they can join a person in their depression. To do this, they need the courage to sit in uncertainty (Melnick & Nevis, 2018). They experience paradoxical hope in hopelessness (Roubal & Řiháček, 2016), in the words of one therapist-research participant: *"Even if I don't see that hope, I hope to see it again."*

Self-Compassion

In his synthesis of neuroscientific and psychotherapeutic knowledge, Siegel (2010) presents the universally recognized example of pre-flight instructions, which inform passengers that it is necessary to first put on their own oxygen masks before helping others. In psychotherapy, this figuratively translates as the necessity of therapists to first develop their own self-understanding and self-compassion. The therapist's self-care can be considered a "prerequisite for the practice of psychotherapy" (Wolf, Goldfried & Muran, 2013, p. 276). Carl Rogers' advice: "You can't help anyone without risking yourself" (in Anderson, 1997, p. 85), can therefore be supplemented with a second part: And you also can't help anyone without taking care of yourself. "Compassion is not only a sensitivity to the client's suffering, it is also a sensitivity to one's own suffering in order to understand the interaction that creates the psychotherapeutic relationship" (Wolf, Goldfried & Muran, 2013, p. 5).

As therapists, using the model presented here to understand our own experience working with depressed clients can help us be kind to ourselves. We can then understand our own experiences of powerlessness, exhaustion and hopelessness as an experiential movement toward the client. A movement that strengthens the therapeutic relationship as a necessary basis of psychotherapeutic work. Conversely, we can understand our experiences of impatience, anger and frustration as an experiential movement away from the client. This allows us to attend to our own needs and bring an alternative perspective to the client in therapy.

Note

1 Quotes come from therapists – research participants. For the sake of readability, I do not provide their identification here for individual statements.

Bibliography

Anderson, H. (1997). *Conversation, language, and possibilities: A postmodern approach to therapy*. Basic Books.

Melnick, J., Nevis, S. M. (2018). *The evolution of the Cape Cod model: Gestalt conversations, theory, and practice*. Gestalt Therapy Book Series, Istituto di Gestalt HCC Italy Publ.

Roubal, J., Řiháček, T. (2016). Therapists' in-session experiences with depressive clients: A grounded theory. *Psychotherapy Research*, 26(2), 206–219.

Siegel, D. J. (2010). *The mindful therapist*. W. W. Norton and Company.

Tartt, D. (2013). *The Goldfinch*. Little, Brown, p. 712.

Wolf, A. W., Goldfried, M. R., Muran, J. C. (2013). Introduction. In Wolf, A. W., Goldfried, M. R., Muran, J. C (Eds.), *Transforming negative reactions to clients: From frustration to compassion*. American Psychological Association, 269–282.

Chapter 5

What Do We Actually Do?

So it seems that as therapists we need to make a "turn to the client" in our minds so that we do not repeat the same relational pattern that the depressed person encounters in other relationships. With this turn, we hope to escape from the absorbing interpersonal pattern in which we ourselves participate in strengthening the depressive dynamics of the contact. For this radical turnaround, where we stop trying to alleviate the client's depression and instead are with them, we need to rewire our minds. It is like switching from one program to another in our minds. But where do we switch from? And where to?

Now we need to return once more and in more detail to the various concepts of psychotherapeutic change as presented in the previous chapter. We will focus on the role of the therapist. What does a therapist do in psychotherapy and why? The answers vary according to different conceptions of psychotherapeutic change.[1]

In the concept of psychotherapeutic change, there have been several shifts in the history of Gestalt therapy, which can also be observed in other psychotherapeutic approaches. At first, the psychology of an individual based on the classical paradigm dominated. Gestalt therapists developed a therapeutic approach that supported change in the client. Such change was conceived within the frame of humanistic tradition as the client's growth as a person.

Parallel to this mono-personal perspective, which still has its place in Gestalt therapy due to its comprehensibility and practicality, the influence of the bi-personal perspective based on the psychology of two (or more) persons grounded in the postmodern paradigm grew stronger. The dialogic approach has become dominant in Gestalt therapy in the last 30 years or so. In this approach, we observe change not in the client's person, but in the therapeutic relationship. Therefore, therapists developed an approach that can support the transformation of relational patterns.

In the nascent development of Gestalt therapy, there was another, radically different theory of change, which this book will try to illustrate. It derives from the perspective of field theory, which has developed and gained consistency over time in Gestalt therapy. Now it seems to play an increasingly important role in the development of the Gestalt therapy approach. We could perhaps say that the use of the field theory perspective in clinical situations is becoming an area that significantly advances the whole approach of contemporary Gestalt therapy.

DOI: 10.4324/9781003500148-6

Each of the three aforementioned perspectives gives us a different kind of understanding and offers different types of guidelines for our work. Each can be useful at different stages of the therapy process. At any given moment, one perspective may become figural while the others retreat into the background. Later, their influence can shift. At the beginning of therapy, for example, the mono-personal perspective is usually in the foreground (the client needs to deal with their troubles), and only after a while does the therapeutic relationship become figural. Each perspective answers these questions differently: What changes in psychotherapy? How can we understand psychopathological symptoms? What kind of change are we moving toward in therapy? How can a therapist support change?

The Mono-Personal Perspective

We observe the person sitting before us to see how they are, how they live. We use a phenomenological method of observation, where we push aside our efforts to change anything. We just observe and respect what appears. We can look at a client like at a sunset (Zinker, 1977). (When watching a sunset, we also don't think it should be a little less red or a little further to the right of that tree…). We use a phenomenological method of observation to capture what is obvious and what is available, both in fixed patterns and in the potential for change. Both are present in the situation here and now.

From this point of view, psychopathology is not a description of a client's dysfunction as a person. It is the therapist's attempt to describe the suffering that the client is experiencing and that is tied to a certain situation and context (Robine, 2011; Salonia, 2007; Gecele & Francesetti, 2007). This suffering stems from a loss of flexibility and creativity in the present situation, when rigid patterns of perception and response *(fixed gestalt)* prevent a person from having satisfying contact with their environment. Psychopathology therefore describes certain fixed patterns of relating to the environment and to oneself, which do not allow the client to use well the available resources and, as a result, to grow. Psychopathological symptoms then represent phenomenologically observable manifestations of such rigid patterns.

In simple terms, we can consider a flexible, creative way of functioning as healthy. By contrast, we can consider a rigid, stereotyped way of functioning as pathological. However, the situation is more complex, because while the first way allows the organism to develop naturally, the second way provides it with security. In a client's personal history the rigid pattern originally represented creative adjustment. It allowed the client to deal with a difficult situation in the best possible way, considering the currently available sources of support. This fixed pattern continues to serve the client as a safe, albeit not fully satisfactory, way of functioning.

From the perspective of Gestalt therapy, there is a continuum without a clear dividing line between healthy and so-called pathological experience. Attempts at diagnostic categorization and nosology in psychotherapy have therefore been viewed with great caution throughout the history of Gestalt therapy (Perls, Hefferline & Goodman, 1951). Instead of clinical classification, the Gestalt therapeutic approach emphasizes the importance of the present situation "here and now." In this way, it attempts to transcend the dichotomy of health versus illness by focusing on the process of an organism making contact with its environment and examining its unique characteristics in a given situation. Focusing on the ever changing present experience enables the client's flexibility and creativity to be brought to life in each unique situation. They can then have the experience of fresh and nourishing contact. The intention is to foster the development and healthy growth of the organism (Perls, Hefferline & Goodman, 1951).

Thus, we use a mono-personal perspective to capture the habitual ways of functioning that served as creative adjustments to help the client survive in difficult circumstances and help them feel safe. At the same time, we support the client in discovering new possibilities available to them and in awakening their potential for growth. The general aim of therapy is to increase the client's ability to creatively adapt to changing life conditions.

We do not perceive psychopathological symptoms as something dysfunctional needing to be fixed. Rather, we see them as an initially useful coping strategy, which later in life limits a person due to its rigidity and inhibits creative adaptations to new conditions. Therapy helps the client find and practice new possibilities of creative adjustment.

We could say that a therapist works like a gardener. They do not generate growth themselves, they do not pull the plant to grow faster. Rather, if we extend the metaphor, they water by providing support and clear the way to sunlight by raising awareness. The therapist-as-gardener respects the client's capacity and pace. We help clients realize how they function in their lives. By becoming aware of fixed patterns, clients are able to use these patterns consciously, or to change them. Thanks to this, they can live their lives more freely and responsibly. We help them find creative new ways of functioning to expand their choices.

The therapist helps the client expand awareness in a special kind of contact that is unusually both supportive for the client and at the same time brings unexpected challenges. We accept and support the client as a person, while at the same time challenging their fixed patterns.

Bi-Personal Perspective

Now we shift our focus from the person sitting in front of us to our relationship with them. We focus on what is happening between us. We focus on the dynamics of the relationship here and now, which is co-created by the client and the therapist. In this relationship, recurring relational patterns come to life, which are then directly available for phenomenological examination. These patterns come alive with the participation of both client and therapist. Thus, we therapists also examine our own reactions as our contribution to the mutual relationship and its form. The therapeutic relationship also allows clients to have a new relational experience with us. This opens up the possibility for them to experience themselves in a new way. Clients can then transfer this new relational experience to their other relationships.

From a bi-personal perspective, experience cannot be attributed exclusively to either the organism or the surrounding environment (Perls, Hefferline & Goodman, 1951; Spagnuolo Lobb, 2003). Rather, we could say that experience emerges from the constantly changing interaction between the individual and the environment. In this way, experience defined as psychopathology also emerges in a relationship. From this point of view, psychopathology is the pathology of a relationship, which a person sensitively perceives as subjective pain and expresses it creatively using psychopathological symptoms (Francesetti, Gecele & Roubal, 2013).

We can therefore see psychopathological symptoms as an individual expression of a specific relational experience. These experiences are missing something essential, for example safety, support or closeness. The relationship suffers due to a specifically modified way of contacting, which does not allow for mutually satisfying fulfillment of the needs of the organism and its environment (Francesetti, Gecele & Roubal, 2013). At the same time, however, this restrictive way of contact deserves appreciation for permitting the organism to survive a relational experience in which the other was not present as needed.

We can then see psychopathological symptoms as a trace of the missing other (Francesetti, 2019a, 2021; Francesetti & Roubal, 2020). This trace comes to life in the present relationship, actualizing itself in the here and now. Relational suffering manifests itself in an individual in their current experience and can also be transformed through this experience (Philippson, 2001). That which was missing manifests in therapy as a need for a new experience in contact with the environment. We can see psychopathological symptoms as an expression of a desire for change, that is, for a relationship in which these symptoms would no longer be needed (Sichera, in Francesetti & Roubal, 2020). Psychopathology thus includes a relational focus on *the next*, toward which it is directed and which gives it meaning (Polster & Polster, 1973; Salonia, 1989; Spagnuolo Lobb, 2003, 2013).

Psychopathological suffering results from a lack of meaningful and fulfilling contact. The relationship suffers and the client shows this in their symptoms. In their story, the client experiences this with the people around them, and it is repeated in the relationship with the therapist. If we understand psychopathology as a manifestation of relational suffering, it seems clear that the psychopathology present in the therapeutic situation must grow out of the suffering of the here-and-now relationship with the therapist. There is no other relationship at that moment. The therapist is the one who is present with the client in the current moment and who also represents the client's general experience with other people.

The therapist is therefore part of the psychopathology that comes to life in the present relationship. They even co-create this psychopathology by their participation in the relationship with the client. The bi-personal perspective offers us a direct possibility of change here. Both therapist and client can become aware of how they contribute to the co-creation of the psychopathology within their mutual relationship. This helps them to consciously step out of a fixed relationship pattern. And this can open up a chance for a new relational experience.

When working from a bi-personal perspective, the therapist stops treating symptoms and encounters the person. Change happens at the relational level between client and therapist. A new healing relational experience is created in which symptoms may no longer be needed. The client feels accepted as they are. Thanks to this experience, they can learn to accept themselves. This gives space for actualizing the client's human potential. The client changes as a person. They become more of who they really are.

How can we as therapists support such change? Change is basically made possible by our availability and willingness to engage in dialogue as a human being. As a person in contact with another person. The client has a chance to be more genuine with us. By being in a pure, honest and open relationship with the client, we open up the opportunity for them to try out new ways of relating. In the bi-personal perspective, what we do as therapists is no longer as important as it was in the mono-personal perspective. Who we become for each other comes to the foreground.[2]

Instead of the gardener metaphor we used with the mono-personal perspective, we can now use the metaphor of a dance (Knijff, 2000; Jacobs, 2020; Philippson, 2019). Both client and therapist are used to operating in certain ways in relationships, and they naturally repeat this respective way in the therapeutic relationship as well. We can imagine this repetition of habitual relational patterns as an old dance, i.e. the way that the body automatically begins to move when music is playing. The old dance of the client meets the old dance of the therapist, both repeating what they are used to (the therapist perhaps with less anxiety about deviating from the habitual).

In a therapeutic situation, client and therapist are condemned to dance together. Yes, condemned. Neither can step out of the therapeutic relationship and stop dancing. When they try, they only change the form of the dance, and in all likelihood they just accentuate their habitual pattern. So they dance together as best they can. Sometimes they step on each other's toes and sometimes they fail to balance a spin because they are standing too far apart.

However, because they have a chance to sensitively perceive and reflect on how they "dance" together in the therapeutic relationship, it is not just a repetition of the "old dance." In order to stay in contact with each other, not lose each other and at the same time not step on each other's toes too much, they need to adapt to a common dance in the here and now situation. This creates creative "new steps." This is a new way of relating that was not planned, that deviates from the usual register and serves to build a living relationship. This metaphor helps us therapists not to push for any particular kind of change, but rather to welcome the change that emerges in a real and humanly honest dialogue.

Field Theory Perspective

To take the field theory perspective, we need to let our mind go wild in a way, allow it to step out of its habitual ways of functioning.[3] We need to observe the situation in a specific way that allows us, above all, to perceive processes. Like when we look at a river and perceive it as a constant movement, which, although imperceptible, is the basic essence of the river. Water that does not flow is no longer a river. Although we cannot capture the flow of the river with our individual senses, in a relaxed state we can tune into it holistically, feel the "rivering."

We can "look" at people, events and ourselves in much the same way as we would at flowing water, at the wind, at movement. To do so, we need to abandon various concepts, namely that of the individual, of objects and of the system of relations between them, as well as the concepts of causality and the linear course of time. Everything flows, everything intertwines; everything is a function of an ongoing process. If from the mono-personal perspective the therapist worked as a gardener and from the bi-personal perspective participated in a therapeutic relational dance, from the field theory perspective both client and therapist are carried along by the flow, that is, by the forces of the field that transcend them. As if they are sailing together on a raft. They can regulate the course of the voyage, but they cannot move or stop the river.

From the field theory perspective, we do not consider the situation to be co-created by therapist and client. The therapeutic situation[4] in its entirety is more than just the interaction of people who meet (Wollants, 2008). The whole is more than the sum of its parts, and here we focus on the more. We can also use the concept of atmosphere as "something we can clearly feel, even if we cannot define and explain it" (Francesetti & Griffero, 2019, p. 1). Atmosphere is "a colloquial expression meaning 'something more' and strongly depends on the context… a feeling or impression that does not belong to the individual and is not internal, but is present in the space and gives a certain 'coloring' to the situation that the person present perceives and experientially belongs to" (Francesetti & Griffero, 2019, p. 1). The atmosphere changes in therapy, and we focus on the process of its transformation. We can notice certain patterns, fixed ways in which the field organizes itself. We can follow the process by which the field organizes here and now into the form of the present situation.

From a field theory perspective, we view client and therapist as processes emerging from the flow by which the field is organizing itself at each moment (Robine, 2011, 2016; Philippson, 2009; Spagnuolo Lobb, 2013; Vázquez Bandín, 2016; Roubal, 2019; Francesetti, 2016, 2019b). Both client and therapist are processes constantly evolving from the situation, which is being transformed in such a way that each present moment is directed toward the next (*now for the next*) (Spagnuolo Lobb, 2013). This constant change, the flow of the situation, is governed by its own dynamics and reshapes its participants. They are functions of the field dynamics. It is important to mention that when taking a field theory perspective, we abandon the concept of causality (even circular causality). We abandon the *active-passive* dichotomy.[5] We abandon the notion that the client and the therapist create the present situation, but neither do we reverse causality in the sense that the situation creates the client and the therapist.

The flow of the situation pushes off from the unique reality of the here and now and naturally directs itself to the next moment. The relational needs of the participants give strength and direction to such flow. By doing so, they allow the situation to transition naturally and smoothly to the next here and now. Such natural flow then offers each participant the opportunity to be truly and uniquely present; to meet others in this way and let oneself be freely transformed via experiencing the flow of live contact.

However, such a natural and graceful flow of the current of the situation is usually limited to some extent by the fixed ways of the field organization. In psychopathological situations, the natural flow of the situation is blocked or rather distorted in a specific way, for example in a depressive way. Both client and therapist are functions of the psychopathological dynamics of the situation. Such dynamics force them both into established ways of the field organization as if into a deep riverbed.

We can now look at the client's symptoms as a function of the current situation, which is organized in a psychopathological way. These rigid ways of field organization deaden the client and prevent them from experiencing satisfying contact. Their suffering is embodied as observable psychopathological symptoms. The therapist, through their experience in the situation here and now, also experiences the deadening dynamics, because they themselves are a function of the psychopathological field organization.

At the same time, the constantly changing process of shaping the situation also offers the potential for liberation toward a natural flow. Much like a stream of water hitting an obstacle, it has the potential to flow naturally and gracefully if the obstacle were to disappear or at least be reduced. The suffering of the participants in the situation is therefore an individually felt manifestation of the *intentionality* of the situation toward a natural flow, which does not have enough support to become a reality.

How can a therapist support change? From the field theory perspective, we see that change goes beyond the people involved in the situation. Change is a process with its own dynamics that "uses" the people involved in order to happen. The therapeutic approach is based on the therapist's aesthetic experience (Bloom, 2003; Francesetti, 2012), on their embodied presence in the flow of the situation. The therapist tunes in to the aesthetics of the contact and lets it guide them. This means that they rely on the clues that come to them through their senses and that guide them in the direction of forming a good whole (*Gestalt*). This method of orientation is based on an intuitive assessment of the situation with the client. It is a specific way of recognizing that appears during contact when the organism and the environment are not yet differentiated (Roubal, Francesetti & Gecele, 2017). Aesthetic knowledge is therefore unspoken and even unnamed. It precedes reflection itself, because it takes place pre-verbally on a corporeal level.

The therapist navigates in the forces of the field by following clues that emerge from perceiving the situation as a whole.[6] As if the therapist and the client were being carried by the power of the river, which is powerful beyond human strength. Whether the river flows fast, swirls in a whirlpool, or stands almost still and is visibly motionless, the client and therapist perceive the river's movement through their experiences. The way they are present is part of a movement that transcends them. A therapist needs to respect and accept this in their work.

The therapist tunes in to the intentionality of the situation (Spagnuolo Lobb, 2013; Francesetti & Roubal, 2013), i.e. to the inclination toward a naturally subsequent moment directed to a meaning-filled process. This process has so far been trapped in the psychopathological field organization. The therapist lends themselves, their embodied being, so that the field forces can materialize. The way the therapist is present in the situation can create an opportunity for what is possible to become actual.

Our main task then is not to hinder this nascent movement. Not to get in the way by having an idea, a vision, an expectation of what should come. The process of change finds itself a path in the unique arrangement of the present situation. It is a path we cannot plan, arrange or even foresee. Change simply happens and we embrace it in whatever form it takes.

From this point of view, we therapists do not cause change or create it together with the client. We just open the door for it. If we do a good job of not blocking its way, the field dynamic can begin to break free, change can begin to happen and the situation can transform. Both client and therapist, who are functions of the field, can transform as well.

Fortunately, in our delicate task of aesthetic attunement to the intentionality of the situation, we find great support in the concept of the paradoxical theory of change (Beisser, 1970). When we stop trying to achieve change, change will come in its own way. During therapy, we can repeat a mantra to ourselves: it's not about what I do, but about how I am present with the client. This can free us therapists from the tasks and demands that we perceive the client placing on us and that we place on ourselves.

The essence of the paradoxical theory of change is that the therapist has no ambition to change what appears as a figure in the present situation. The therapist, by transforming their way of being in the situation, enables the transformation of background processes, from which the transformed figure emerges. "Nature heals and the doctor entertains the patient in the meantime." This saying of Voltaire's, commonplace in the Czech Republic, could also apply to psychotherapy. If we try to help the client, we risk getting in the way of the natural healing processes. In helping, we are likely promoting our own idea of what the client should be like.

Perhaps we could even say that as therapists we are paid for what we do not do. We are trained to tame our instinctual helping responses and to be in a therapeutic situation without direction or expectation. We are paid to withstand our powerless-ness and remain truly and freely present. When we transform our way of being with the client in this way, the possibility of transforming the whole situation opens up. The situation itself can begin to liberate itself. Distorted fixed processes can start to loosen and redirect themselves to free the potential of the situation for the natural field dynamic, whatever form it may take.

Theoretical Understanding as Support for Therapists

Understanding what takes place in therapy and the role of the therapist in such a process can serve the therapist as a source of self-support in challenging clinical situations. It is important not to confuse the theory of change with the change itself.

The theory of change represents our understanding and offers useful guidelines for therapeutic work. In the face of the change itself, we must humbly admit the limitations of our theory.

Basically, the theory of the psychotherapeutic process does not tell us what really happens. Rather, it says there is a way of understanding what happens. We can lean on that, stay calm even in challenging situations, be freely and truthfully present, let go of expectations and hold on to hope. Forget the theory and be ready to sit down with the other and encounter one another.

However, our understanding stays with us implicitly because it has established how we are with the other. We can be with the depressed person like a gardener, watering the depression with support and letting the change grow. We can be with them as a dance partner who is aware that depression is co-created here and now in the relationship with the client, and that change will come in the creative new steps that arise from the dancers' mutual contact. Or we can be on a raft with the client. We steer a bit, but sometimes the raft spins around and the client steers a bit. We need the client to row where we cannot reach. Together we try to sail through the rapids by making use of the current, which carries us along with the client through the depressing way.

Illustrative Case Study

Vojta came to therapy with insomnia and abdominal pain. The somatic doctors found nothing they could treat and referred him to psychotherapy. Early in psychotherapy, we realized that the symptoms of insomnia and abdominal pain were the most visible manifestations of general exhaustion, which included chronic fatigue, headaches, obesity-related overeating, and long-term depressive moods.

Vojta attended therapy for seven months and then, before the summer break, he recapitulated what had changed for him: "My sleeping is still bad, but it is true that my stomach hurts less. I know what to watch out for more." (Not a very flattering result for a therapist after such a long stretch of therapy. The symptoms that had bothered the client, which had brought him to therapy, and which he wanted to change, had not changed at all or only partially.)

"But mainly other things have changed. Well, actually I lost my job... and now my wife and I have really started arguing a lot, sometimes it looks like divorce is on the way." (So changes are happening in other areas than those in which the client had wanted to see change. And they are not exactly what the client imagined before entering therapy.)

Therapist: "When you sum it up like that, I'm wondering if you actually find therapy helpful and if you even want to continue after the holidays?"

"Yeah, I do."

"Could you expand on why you want to continue?"

"Well, I don't know exactly. I don't really understand what is happening to me in my life. But I have the feeling that it somehow makes sense to me, even though

it's all in motion. And mostly, I see that you are calm, so, it probably means something, right?" (This is a key message from the client. By being "calm," the therapist provides support, motivation and hope to the client. But how to stay calm? This is where the theory of change will serve as an anchor for the therapist, as a reminder not to panic, even if the change is not exactly as expected.)

To understand the process of change in therapy with Vojta, we need to see the bigger picture. At the beginning of therapy, Vojta recognized the most significant source of stress in his life: his current job and, above all, his despotic boss. Later, he also saw how much the boss resembled his father, a professional soldier who had died six years earlier. He always let his father dictate things and even chose his current profession according to his father's wishes. The experience with his father shaped him significantly; he learned to live life according to the expectations of others, whom he placed in a position of authority.

In therapy, he gradually discovered that at the age of 39 it was about time to emancipate himself. He began to express his opinions, which led to conflicts at work and eventually to his dismissal. Vojta then worked in several other jobs, which never lasted long. Basically, he was trying to find something of his own, to make his own choices. But this was difficult for him partly because he had not yet learned how. And also because it led him to a more general search for what he actually wanted to do with his life. And to existential doubts about his purpose in this world. While he was dealing with such questions, his wife was getting impatient because the family – they had two children in elementary school – was running out of money. In addition, Vojta stopped being accommodating no matter what and began to delineate himself even vis-à-vis his wife, which led to arguments that were surprising and painful for them both. At the same time, it also revived their relationship, especially sexually. They truly loved each other, thus there was hope that weathering the current crisis could enrich their marriage.

It therefore seemed comprehensible to the therapist that the symptoms that brought Vojta to therapy were related to his pattern of living according to the expectations of others and to the resulting stress. In therapy, Vojta began to realize and gradually change this automatic pattern of behavior. Creating a new way of relating to the people around you and to yourself takes place through searching, trying and learning from failures. According to the therapist, Vojta is now in this stage of the therapeutic process.

This particular case's theory of change, as described above, served the therapist as a supportive third party, a hand to hold when doubts loomed large. These doubts were of an existential nature, were a prominent feature of the given situation and were strongly perceived by the client as well. The therapist's own conceptualization of the process of change in psychotherapy allowed them to remain calmly present and available to the client. This support enabled the client to persevere through the difficult phase of the therapeutic process and to continue therapy.

To illustrate the three perspectives described earlier, we will now briefly look at one aspect of the therapeutic process: how Vojta handles his own needs. To give a more detailed idea, we will look at one specific therapeutic situation and explore the possible ways of working with it based on the different perspectives.[7]

Mono-personal perspective

In his childhood, Vojta did not have the support to learn to recognize his own needs and to be able to confidently enter into contact with his environment with the intention of fulfilling his needs. Instead, he creatively adapted to a difficult situation and learned to both read and meet the needs of others very well. In short: he turned the impulses to fulfill his own needs back toward himself (retroflexion) and projected his needs onto others (projection).

> *At one point during the seventeenth session, Vojta speaks quietly, looks at the ground and breathes very shallowly. Therapist: "Could you just focus on your breathing for a moment?"*
>
> *"I'm actually barely breathing..."*
>
> *"And what is it like?"*
>
> *"I don't know... unpleasant. I don't have the strength for anything."*
>
> *"Ah... you don't have the strength for anything... Well, what do you need right now?"*
>
> *"I don't know... nothing I guess... you think that..."*
>
> *"Hmm... and what does your body need?"*
>
> *"Well, to take a breath, that's obvious. But I'm not doing it for some reason... weird..."*
>
> *"What do you find weird?"*
>
> *"That I need something and I still don't do it."*

The therapist's support offers Vojta a path to increased self-awareness, which gradually helps him to recognize his own repeating pattern. In the further course of therapy, he accepts responsibility for this pattern and gradually frees himself from it. Instead, he learns an alternative: to notice bodily signals related to his own needs and to use the impulse associated with bodily discomfort to act. As Vojta declares after a while: *"When I have trouble breathing, I straighten up. Yes, I also mean it figuratively."*

Bi-personal perspective

After his formative experience with paternal authority, Vojta automatically takes a subordinate, obedient position toward others. From a bi-personal perspective, we do not attribute the phenomena mentioned above (projection of needs onto others and retroflexion of impulses to fulfill needs) to the client, but understand them as co-created by the client and the therapist.

> *Vojta speaks quietly, looks at the ground and breathes very shallowly. Therapist: "Could you tell me how you feel here, with me, now?"*

"What? ... well, normal..."
"I noticed you're barely breathing."
"Yeah, well... I..., yeah, you're right, I'm not breathing."
"Is there anything I can do to make it easier for you to breathe with me?"
"What? ... That's a weird question... I mean, I apologize."
"How is your breathing now?"
"It's better... How did you do that?"
  "I don't know, somehow we did it together... Do you have any idea how that could have happened?"

The fundamentally important part in therapy now takes place on a relational level. On the one hand, Vojta and the therapist slip into a habitual pattern, where Vojta submits and the therapist acts from the position of authority. On the other hand, Vojta has the opportunity to create a new relationship experience with an authority who is interested in his opinion and is willing to adapt to his needs. Such repeated experience with the therapist in the course of therapy leads to Vojta's greater self-confidence and the courage to define himself in contact with others.

Field theory perspective

We see insensitivity to one's own needs and retroflexion as field phenomena that transcend both the client as an individual and the client's relationship with the therapist. These phenomena reveal how the field is being organized. Both client and therapist are a function of the field organization at the given moment, as if they were being swept along by the current of the situation.

Vojta speaks quietly, looks at the ground and breathes very shallowly. The therapist notices this and then shifts his focus from the client back to himself, to his experience of the here and now, especially his own body. He realizes that he isn't breathing freely either, sitting slightly forward in his chair and trying to figure out a good way to work with such a subdued client. He realizes he has placed a demand on himself: to find a good way to work with this client. With this demand, he makes himself less free, he limits himself. So he leans back in his chair, inhales and exhales, relaxes. He lets go of the demands he made on himself and anchors himself with his feet firmly on the ground. He then feels freer, looks at Vojta, smiles with relief.
  Vojta looks at him questioningly, then looks back at the ground. After a moment of silence, he turns to the therapist: "You know, I actually wanted to talk to you about something else today..." He speaks louder and looks at the therapist more often. The change in topic and method of communication is clear. What's also clear is that Vojta is now breathing more deeply.

By transforming their way of being in the situation, the therapist opens up the possibility for the field to be organized in a new way. A new figure can emerge from the transformed background. The therapist does not try to change Vojta or their relationship. Accepting the situation as it is opens up the possibility for change.

We see how each different perspective highlights a distinct aspect of the therapeutic process and engenders a change in the way of working. The three perspectives described above are used in this book to describe what happens with depression in psychotherapy, and how the therapist experiences the situation with the depressed client. These are the dynamics of the depressive functioning of the client, the dynamics of the co-creation of depression and the dynamics of the depressive situation as such. We will focus mostly on the field theory perspective, which brings significant new inspirations to psychotherapeutic work in the field of psychopathology.

Notes

1 The following overview shows these different concepts using the example of Gestalt therapy, but therapists following other approaches will probably also find parallels here.
2 In order to remain in the position from which we encounter the other person, without trying to change their symptoms, the principles of the dialogical approach (Jacobs, 1995; Yontef, 2005) can help us: inclusion, confirmation, presence and surrendering to dialogue.
3 The processes I am trying to describe here are pre-verbal, experienced bodily and perceived synesthetically (without distinguishing individual senses). These are processes that happen even before self-environment differentiation (see Francesetti & Roubal (2020) for more details) and that belong to the situation and not to the individual. That is why their linguistic description is very difficult or impossible, and why perhaps we can come closest to understanding them through metaphors. I thus ask the reader for tolerance and creative reading.
4 The concept of a "situation" is derived from field theory. A situation represents a temporally and spatially defined process of field organization here and now. However, the concept of a situation varies among authors depending on their conception of field theory (Wollants, 2008; Robine, 2011; Spagnuolo Lobb, 2013; Francesetti, 2015; Francesetti & Roubal, 2020).
5 Perls, Hefferline, and Goodman (1951) instead speak of a *"middle mode,"* a natural spontaneity that transcends (and includes) activity and passivity.
6 Francesetti refers to Aristotle and elaborates that the therapist navigates by means of *phronesis* (Francesetti, 2019a; Francesetti & Roubal, 2020), i.e. the wisdom that appears in the totality of the situation itself. We use different kinds of orientation in different situations. For example, when driving a car, we know how the car works and what the rules of the road are *(epistemological knowledge)*. We know what to do to control the car *(technical knowledge)*. But when we need to know when and how much to slow down in a turn, we rely on our perception of the whole situation in the present moment *(phronetic knowledge)*.
7 Here are three variants of how the therapy could have proceeded. One of them actually happened and the other two are hypothetical, derived from other real situations with clients in order to illustrate the different ways of working based on understanding the therapeutic situation from different perspectives (in the sense of a composite case study (Gabbard, 2000)). It is deliberately not said which of the possibilities actually happened, so that it is not favored, because all three perspectives and the interventions derived from them have their place in Gestalt therapy.

Bibliography

Beisser, A. (1970). The paradoxical theory of change. In Fagan, J., Shepherd, L. (Ed.), *Gestalt Therapy Now*. Harper Colophon Books, 77–80.

Bloom, D. J. (2003). Tiger! tiger! burning bright. Aesthetic values as clinical values in Gestalt therapy. In Spagnuolo, M. L., Amendt-Lyon N. (Eds.), *Creative license: The art of Gestalt therapy*. Springer Verlag, 63–78.

Francesetti, G. (2012). Pain and beauty: From psychopathology to the aesthetics of contact. *British Gestalt Journal*, 21(2), 4–18.

Francesetti, G. (2015). From individual symptoms to psychopathological fields: Towards a field perspective on clinical human suffering. *British Gestalt Journal*, 24(1), 5–19.

Francesetti, G. (2016). "You cry, I feel pain:" The emerging, co-created self as the foundation of anthropology, psychopathology and treatment in Gestalt therapy. In Robine, J. M. (Ed.), *Self: A polyphony of contemporary Gestalt therapists*. L'Exprimerie.

Francesetti, G. (2019a). The field strategy in clinical practice: Towards a theory of therapeutic phronesis." In Brownell, P. (Ed.), *Handbook for theory, research and practice in Gestalt therapy* (2nd ed.). Cambridge Scholars Publishing, 268–302.

Francesetti, G. (2019b). A clinical exploration of atmospheres: Towards a field-based clinical practice. In Francesetti, G. A., Griffero T. (Eds.), *Psychopathology and atmospheres: Neither inside nor outside*. Cambridge Scholars Publishing, 35–68.

Francesetti, G. (2021). *Fundamentals of phenomenological-Gestalt psychopathology: A light introduction*. L'Exprimerie.

Francesetti, G., Griffero, T. (2019). Introduction. In Francesetti, G., Griffero, T. (Eds.), *Neither inside nor outside: Psychopathology and atmospheres*. Cambridge Scholars Publishing, 1–5.

Francesetti, G., Roubal, J. (2013) Gestalt therapy approach to depressive experiences. In Francesetti, G., Gecele, M., Roubal, J. (Eds.), *Gestalt therapy in clinical practice: From psychopathology to the aesthetics of contact*. Franco Angeli, 433–494.

Francesetti, G., Roubal, J. (2020). Field theory in contemporary Gestalt therapy, Part 1: Modulating the therapist's presence in clinical practice. *Gestalt Review*, 24(2), 113–136.

Francesetti, G., Gecele, M., Roubal, J. (2013). Gestalt therapy approach to psychopathology. In Francesetti, G., Gecele, M., Roubal, J. (Eds.), *Gestalt therapy in clinical practice: From psychopathology to the aesthetics of contact*. FrancoAngeli. 59–76.

Gabbard, G. O. (1999). *Countertransference issues in psychiatric treatment*. American Psychiatric Press.

Gecele, M., Francesetti, G. (2007). The polis as the ground and horizon of therapy. In Francesetti, G. (Ed.), *Panic attacks and postmodernity: Gestalt therapy between clinical and social perspective*. FrancoAngeli, 170–212.

Jacobs, L. (1995). Dialogue in Gestalt theory and therapy. In Hycner, R., Jacobs, L. (Eds.), *The healing relationship in Gestalt therapy*. Gestalt Journal Press, 51–84.

Jacobs, L. (2020). Engaged surrender: The polarity of dialogue in Gestalt therapy. *Gestalt Review*, 24(2), 163–177.

Knijff, E. (2000). *De therapeut als clown, randopmerkingen van een Gestalttherapeut*. EPO.

Perls, F., Hefferline, R. F., Goodman, P. (1951). *Gestalt therapy: Excitement and growth in the human personality*. Julian Press.

Philippson, P. (2001). *Self in relation*. Karnac Books.

Philippson, P. (2009). *The emergent self: An existential-Gestalt approach*. Karnac Books.

Philippson, P. (2019). *We can be together, but you and me can meet* (Topics in Gestalt Therapy Book 4). Kindle Edition, www.amazon.co.uk/Together-Meet-Topics-Gestalt-Therapy-ebook/dp/B06Y1D2X14/ref=sr_1_12?keywords=philippson&qid=1557160100&s=digital-text&sr=1-12

Polster, E., Polster, M. (1973) *Gestalt therapy integrated, contours of theory and practice*. Brunner/Mazel.

Robine, J. M. (2011). *On the occasion of an other.* Gestalt Journal Press.

Robine, J. M. (2016). *Self, a polyphony of contemporary Gestalt therapists.* L'Exprimerie.

Roubal, J. (2019). Theory of change. In Francesetti, G., Vázquez Bandín, C., Reed, E. (Eds.), *Obsessive-compulsive experiences: A Gestalt therapy.* Los Libros del CTP, 9–20.

Roubal, J., Francesetti, G., Gecele, M. (2017). Aesthetic diagnosis in Gestalt therapy. *Behavioral Sciences*, 7(4). doi: 10.3390/bs7040070.

Salonia, G. (1989). From we to I-thou: A contribution to an evolutive theory of contact. *Studies in Gestalt Therapy*, 1, 31–42.

Salonia, G. (2007). Social changes and psychological disorders: Panic attacks in postmodernity. In Francesetti, G. (Ed.), *Panic attacks and postmodernity: Gestalt therapy between clinical and social perspectives.* FrancoAngeli.

Spagnuolo Lobb, M. (2003). Creative adjustment in madness: A Gestalt therapy model for seriously disturbed patients. In Spagnuolo Lobb, M., Amendt-Lyon, N. (Eds.), *Creative license, the art of Gestalt therapy.* Springer, 25–31.

Spagnuolo Lobb, M. (2013). *The now-for-next in psychotherapy: Gestalt therapy recounted in post-modern society.* FrancoAngeli.

Vázquez Bandín, C. (2016) In *Self: A Polyphony of Gestalt Therapists.* Edited by J.-M. Robine. L'Exprimeire.

Wells, B. (2018). *The end of loneliness.* Sceptre, p. 123.

Wollants, G. (2008). *Gestalt therapy: Therapy of the situation.* Sage.

Yontef, G. (2005). Gestalt therapy theory of change. In Woldt, A., Toman, S. (Eds.), *Gestalt therapy: History, theory, and practice.* Sage, 81–100.

Zinker, J. (1977). *Creative process in Gestalt therapy.* Brunner-Mazel.

Chapter 6

Letting Pain Be Felt

In depression, suffering consists of a deep pain of the soul and at the same time a general inhibition, which protects against fully experiencing the pain (Francesetti & Roubal, 2013). The ability to reduce awareness of the excruciating pain is a creative adjustment that allows a person to go on living. However, the same ability prevents that person from living fully. It inhibits them from perceiving the vibrancy of contact with their environment, entering it as themselves and experiencing themselves changing in this contact. All of this is extremely difficult, if not impossible, in depression. That is why a depressed person is so painfully alone in their suffering.

If this is how we understand the suffering of depressed clients, it leads us to a paradoxical approach when working with them. In psychotherapy, we do not help alleviate pain, but rather allow the client to go through the pain. Our intention is to alleviate the suffering of unbearable loneliness. With our presence, we then help clients to begin to feel the pain, begin to feel themselves. To move toward the darkness and pass through it. The support of human contact will allow them to more fully experience the painful present, to start living. Our intention is to create a relationship in which there is no longer the need to protect oneself from pain, to deaden oneself. To offer the client a relationship in which symptoms of depression are not needed.

The depressive vicious circle can thus transform into the cleansing pain of grieving. When working with depression, as therapists, we do not help the client to get out from depression, but we assist in stirring up movement in the depths of depression. We help transform a whirlpool of depression into a wave of grief.

Depression and Grieving

In this regard, the distinction between depression and grieving is crucial. Firstly, because we work with each of these experiences differently. And secondly, because the grieving process offers us a way out of depression. Depression can be understood as a disruption or blockage of the natural, cleansing process of grieving.

Although the symptoms of sadness and depression can look very similar, the dynamics of these processes are different (see, for example, Freud, 1917 or Bowlby,

DOI: 10.4324/9781003500148-7

1980).[1] Grieving allows a person to cope with loss.[2] To process the relational experience with the one who has gone. The emptiness left after them shows the depth and value of their presence. The grieving period serves to balance dual loyalties: to the relationship that is no more and to the life that carries on (Francesetti & Roubal, 2013). Grieving thus enables the preservation of what was precious in the past (Cavaleri, in Francesetti & Roubal, 2013) and reconnecting with life in the present again.

When grieving, the inaccessibility of the other comes to the foreground and memories of shared experiences emerge. In this way, the experience of the past relationship is incorporated into the present. The one who remains learns to carry with them the one who is no more. Grieving represents a period of integration of experiencing the "presence of absence" (Francesetti & Roubal, 2013, p. 438). However, it is not only a reflection and processing of the past. It is also a creative time that allows the bereaved to come to terms with who they became with the departed person and who they now become without them.

While the essence of the grieving person's suffering lies in the fact that their loved one is no longer reachable, the experience of depression is different. When experiencing deep depression, what anchored a person and connected them to the world is lost, it is an experience of the "absence of presence" (Francesetti & Roubal, 2013, p. 440). In grieving, one loses the person to whom they were attached. By contrast, in the case of deep depression, what is lost are the conditions that would make such attachment possible.

The severity of the client's depression can then be assessed according to how much they are disconnected from the space "in-between"[3] themselves and their surroundings. In deep depression, the ties that connect a person to the world and life disappear. The living movement by which these bonds are constantly recreated moment by moment disappears. In this lies the uniqueness of the experience of deep depression. The space "in-between" no longer offers meeting, instead it becomes an insurmountable abyss.

From Psychopathology to the Aesthetics of Contact[4]

We sit with the client, watch them and also observe how we ourselves feel with them. It would probably be natural for us to immediately start distinguishing and sorting out individual aspects of the situation. Differentiating whether they are functional or dysfunctional, healthy or unhealthy, flexible or fixed. Such a distinction allows us to orientate ourselves in the clinical situation. It begins to show us where the weak points are, what needs to be changed, what to work on. The psychopathological aspects of the situation naturally attract our attention. And we differentiate them from healthy functioning aspects, that is, sources of support. This process also begins to clarify our role in the specific situation with the client and our task in the here and now.

In this sense, focusing on psychopathology works well, because it helps us calm down, find our place, anchor ourselves. Nevertheless, we pay for such calming down with a certain limitation. By dividing the flow of the present situation into individual aspects, which we then evaluate in a certain way, we limit our ability to perceive the whole. We stop at partial aspects, and thus we miss what additionally appears in the whole situation. We fail to see how the whole is different from the sum of the individual parts.

It can be helpful here to tune into the perception of the "aesthetics of contact." This holistic way of perceiving a situation enables us to use our senses. It is not about evaluating what we think is and is not beautiful. That would bring us back to the evaluation approach. Instead, we perceive the quality of the present experience with our senses. What we perceive, we do not grasp individually, but let it organize into a certain whole. We wait for this whole to become elucidated for us.

Psychotherapy can be seen as a delicate mixture of science and art (Skála, in Vymětal, 2003). Attuning to the aesthetics of contact as therapists, we accentuate this artistic part of our work. We become "artists" in order to perceive the aesthetic qualities of the entirety of the present situation: temperature, structure, mood and the like. We allow ourselves to be surprised by what appears thanks to our sensory perception of the situation and how assembles itself. Such a perception of the situation is very difficult to put into words. Maybe metaphors can help. We can perceive contact with the client, for example, as a path through the fog, from which the dark outlines of unclear objects suddenly emerge and then disappear again. Or we feel like we are on a roller coaster with the client. The important thing is that each such metaphor appears to us anew in each new situation.

In my opinion, the benefit of the aesthetics of contact is that it empowers us to perceive what is otherwise unreachable. In this way, it is as if we tune into a dimension that we cannot perceive directly. We can imagine that this is similar to trying to explain what a cone is to a creature who lives in a two-dimensional world. The flat being will only be able to see a circle or a triangle. But if they are sufficiently sensitive to the situation as a whole, they will feel that out of all the different shapes, this particular circle and this triangle somehow belong together. When they are together, it is as if something extra appears, something qualitatively new. They sense this, even though they have no capacity to see the three-dimensional cone. In this way, perhaps the aesthetics of contact gives us an insight into otherwise invisible connections, contexts and meanings. Thanks to holistic perception, it is as if we can sense the whole in another dimension, which we cannot perceive directly.

As psychotherapists, we experience firsthand psychopathology coming to life in a therapeutic situation. Thanks to our physical presence with the client, we can taste, feel, hear or smell the psychopathological processes by which the psychotherapeutic situation organizes. Through our senses, in an aesthetic way (Perls, Hefferline & Goodman, 1951; Bloom, 2003), we perceive the process of field organization, its grace or disharmony, its flexibility or coldness.

Every situation is unique, we perceive it in a unique way, and thus every therapeutic intervention is a newly created piece of art. We are present to what emerges and also what is missing in the given situation, to *emerging absences* (Francesetti, 2019, 2021; Francesetti & Roubal, 2020). We need to become sensitive to the subtle tones of the ever-changing complexities of our experiences in the client's presence, because within them we can catch a glimpse of the forces needed to transform the psychopathological field.

The Whirlpool of Depression and the Wave of Grief

The therapist's experience is different in the presence of a grieving client and in the presence of a depressed client. With a grieving client, we may experience the weight and constriction of the situation, but we are not likely to experience it as overwhelming or personally threatening to us (as happens with a depressed client). Remaining experientially immersed in a heavy and painful sadness will probably be challenging, but at the same time fulfilling and satisfying. We are usually able to stay in the sharing of grief for as long as the client needs. We do not feel the need to experientially withdraw from the client. The space "in-between" still resonates, albeit darkly, and allows us to connect with the client. We can then not only give, but also reap from lively ongoing contact.

In grieving, we co-experience sadness with the client and at the same time perceive the meaningfulness of what we do. Sadness is an emotion that accompanies the healthy grieving process, and our experience of meaningfulness informs us of this ongoing healing process. We do not try to obstruct it, interfere with it or avoid it. We create a safe space for the client and for ourselves in which it is possible to go through grief and to integrate this experience.

The therapeutic approach with grief is different than with depression. Grieving is a moving process into which we dive together with the client and which also brings us back to the surface. Our support naturally aims toward experiencing the pain together, completing the "tasks of grieving" (Sabar, 2000, p. 152) and processing the experiences associated with loss. As therapists, we are aware of this pain and heaviness. For us, accompanying the client and growing experientially close to them is simply a result of the situation. When descending with the client, we naturally follow the human healer's impulse. We ride down on a wave of grief and descend with the confidence that after sailing through the darkness it will bring us back up to the light.

Here, in contrast, lies the insidiousness of the depressive field. Since it is so similar to grieving in its heaviness and darkness, we are likewise driven by the natural healer's impulse and we thus trustingly begin to delve into the depth of the depressive situation. Only after a while do we discover that in this case, the situation different. We realize we have sunk into a bottomless black hole and cannot rely on the natural healing process of grieving. We cannot ride the wave of grief that would, after experiencing loss, carry us back up into life. With depression, the natural healing process of grieving is disrupted. Our experience of powerlessness and hopelessness lets us know this is a different situation, as does the impression that it is too much for us. That it is dangerous for us personally and instead of a healer's impulse to join, we experience the self-preservation impulse that leads us to abandon the client.

We aesthetically perceive the whirlpool of depression that drags us and the client down. In the case of the client, this movement is clear. They fall into depression[5] and this fall affects all aspects of their life. Mood and energy drop, initiative and joy are lost. Downward movement is characteristic of depression. However, it is not only about moving downward, but also about limiting, narrowing. As already mentioned, a depressed person limits their activities and contacts, narrows their spectrum of coping mechanisms and variety of experiences. As a third defining aspect, in addition to falling and narrowing, there is also looping, or rather, going around in a circle. A person is not able to escape from a depressive way of functioning; they find themselves in a vicious circle of depression. In this circle, the organism's ability to cope with its own mental and physical processes, as well as with external demands, reduces. This leads to a more frequent feeling of failure and tendency to self-blame, which subsequently deepen the depressive state, thus further decreasing the capacity of the organism. When we put together these three types of movement – falling, narrowing and going round in a vicious circle, we get a picture of the whirlpool of depression that pulls the client down and in which we also suddenly find ourselves.

Being no exception, we therapists also succumb to the whirlpool of depression that pulls us into a painfully deserted void. Into a hopelessly deserted void. Like the client, we lose hope when we experience the futility of trying to achieve contact with the other. The space between us does not resonate, does not connect. In interpersonal contact, the usual continuously shared responses of the other, which fill space and time during psychotherapy, are absent. The space "in-between" is a cold void, lacking lively interest or impulse. We feel that the situation is not moving anywhere. As if time slowed down and space dilated. We feel that time almost stops, the session drags on unbearably, movements are slow and laborious, as if we were moving in thick honey. We also perceive the space we are in to be getting bigger. The distance between the therapist's chair and the client's chair seems enormous, even insurmountable. The power required to cover this distance does not seem to be available. There is a chasm between us.

At the same time, the suffering caused by this hopelessly unbridgeable chasm shows us that in the very essence of the depressive situation lies a deep desire for contact with another. That a depressive situation inclines toward contact. The inability to realize this intentionality then causes pain.

The task of us therapists is not to pull the client out of depression, but to help transform the whirlpool of depression into a wave of grief. Our aim is to allow the natural healing process of grieving to be set in motion, whereby the experience of depressive emptiness turns into the pain of sadness and through it to the awareness of unfulfilled needs. The needs of a living, grieving person.

But careful, the sadness must not be skipped. It is fundamentally important to allow ourselves to experience it, as it restarts the grieving process disrupted by depression. The therapist can help this by not running away from their experience of powerlessness and frustration, by staying close to the client and by listening to the intentionality toward contact. Staying within reach is key. There is, after all, only minimal movement in the depressive stillness, when the client occasionally peeks out, just in case someone is around their deserted hopelessness. And then it is important to be within reach, to resonate. At such a moment, it is not our words that matter, but our eyes. At such a moment, the client looks for the eyes of a living person, in which they might catch sight of that tiny spark of hope that brought them to therapy.

Valerie is 59, we are meeting in psychotherapy for the thirteenth time.

"I sit at home, look out the window, I see nothing. Why keep living? It's no use." Her faded eyes, her dry voice, the atmosphere of a funeral parlor. I sit before Valerie, I look at her – and I see nothing. Why am I sitting here anyway? It's no use. I'm already in it, with her. All right then, this is how I feel with her. And thanks to that, I can conjecture how difficult it is for her, what her life is like. She sits in this every day. What does she actually do all day? I would like to know that. Not really, but I would still be a little interested. Better than this funeral parlor atmosphere.

"Hmm... you sit at home and look out the window... Could you tell me what you did today?"

"Total shit! I mean, sorry. I did nothing. Nothing, nothing, nothing."

Well that's quite interesting, suddenly resigned loneliness turns into angry frustration. I probably contributed to it when I asked her a little out of context about what she did today. Which is a good thing, I let myself be led by a pinch of curiosity and what appeared? (Total sh*t.) Anyway, a bit of revival in hopelessness.

"Sorry to pry, I'm really interested. How was your day, what did you do?"

"Yeah, I'm sorry for snapping like that. It's infuriating that I can't manage anything. I don't want anything, I'm not interested in anything, as I'm always at home, I'm weak and I can't even do anything anymore... What did I do today? I stared at the ceiling from three in the morning, then I stared out the window, fed the canary, read leaflets from the mailbox, stared out the window again. That's all. It's useless."

That anger gave her a little strength, she speaks for an unusually long time. But despair is pulling her down again. I've heard this from her so many times. Hopelessness is already pulling me down too. I could feel it as she spoke. A weight fell on my shoulders and my head became empty. I can't think, I don't know what to do next. This has happened so many times. It's useless.

Actually, there was a small glimmer in the heavy grey, something caught my attention, a sign of life when she spoke. The canary! Yes, when she mentioned the canary, it took me aback. I didn't know she had one, she never talked about it. I thought she was all alone at home. And yet there is another living being there! I'm interested in that. Bless, I'm interested in something, so I'll try to go in this direction.

"You fed the canary? You have a canary?"

"Well yeah, I got it from a former colleague at work."

"What colleague?"

"Well, Kamila, she keeps trying to get me hiking, keeps bothering me, I don't answer her calls anymore."

"What does the canary look like?"

"Yellow. It makes a mess, I cover my ears in the morning so I don't hear him. I say to myself, just…"

"Just what?"

"Just die!"

Valerie suddenly bursts into tears. I'm surprised, I wait to see what happens. I settle more consciously in the chair, straighten my back and breathe. I don't know what's coming. I'm ready.

"Hmm."

"I don't know why I'm sobbing here, sorry."

"You started to cry when you said that the canary should just die."

Valerie starts crying again. *"Do you know what came to me at that moment? I felt the same way with my husband. When he was annoying. And then he died."* She cries quietly and blows her nose into a handkerchief.

I sit and breathe. The funeral parlor atmosphere really makes sense now. Now it fits, this is how you cry at a funeral. I feel weight and joy within it. I want to be in this with her.

"Hmm… Will you tell me about him?"

"He was kind of grey, always with me, I'd run away from him to work. And then he died."

Valerie has her hands on her knees, fingers clutching her skirt, head down, shoulders shaking. Tears drip on her skirt.

I sit and breathe. I am with her, I feel joy. I smile a little. Valerie suddenly looks at me, I don't manage to hide my smile in time.

"Well yeah, it's true, I miss him, the grey man. I'd never have thought that would happen."

There is pain and life in her eyes. I look at her with tears in my eyes. I am glad to be with her. And I am grateful to the canary. In the funerary atmosphere, it was like a pointer toward life, all you had to do was follow curiosity.

Notes

1 The therapeutic approach is also different. Working psychotherapeutically in the same way with both grief and depression may even harm the client (Smith, 1985).

2 Here, by way of illustration, we focus on the loss of a close person, but it applies to significant losses of various kinds.

3 Experiences of grieving and deep depression (melancholia) represent extreme forms of depressive experiences, between which there is a scale of fixed, to varying degrees, relational processes, which are manifested by variously ranked depressive experiences.

4 Here I would like to express my deep gratitude for the fruitful and for me personally very enriching collaboration with Gianni Francesetti and Michela Gecele, with whom I collaborated editorially on the book *Gestalt Therapy in Clinical Practice: From Psychopathology to the Aesthetics of Contact* (2013). Much of what I describe here now was born out of our collaboration – my thanks to them both.

5 Etymologically, depression means descent, pressing down, a hollow or a chasm.

Bibliography

Baume, S. (2018). *A line made by walking*. Mariner Books, p. 222.

Bloom, D. J. (2003). Tiger! tiger! burning bright: Aesthetic values as clinical values in Gestalt therapy. In Spagnuolo, M. L., Amendt-Lyon, N. (Eds.), *Creative license: The art of Gestalt therapy*. Springer Verlag.

Bowlby, J. (1980). *Attachment and loss*. Vol. 3: *Loss, sadness and depression*. The Hogarth Press.

Francesetti, G. (2019). The field strategy in clinical practice: Towards a theory of therapeutic phronesis. In Brownell, P. (Ed.), *Handbook for theory, research and practice in Gestalt therapy* (2nd ed.). Cambridge Scholars Publishing, 268–302.

Francesetti, G. (2021). *Fundamentals of phenomenological-Gestalt psychopathology: A light introduction.* L'Exprimerie.

Francesetti, G., Roubal, J. (2013) Gestalt therapy approach to depressive experiences. In Francesetti, G., Gecele, M., Roubal, J. (Eds.), *Gestalt therapy in clinical practice: From psychopathology to the aesthetics of contact*. Franco Angeli, 433–494.

Francesetti, G., Roubal, J. (2020). Field theory in contemporary Gestalt therapy, Part 1: Modulating the therapist's presence in clinical practice. *Gestalt Review*, 24(2), 113–136.

Francesetti G., Gecele, M., Roubal, J. (Eds.) (2013). *Gestalt therapy in clinical practice: From psychopathology to the aesthetics of contact*. Franco Angeli.

Freud, S. (1917). Trauer Und Melancholie. *International Journal of Psychoanalysis*, 4(6), 288–301.

Perls, F., Hefferline, R. F., Goodman, P. (1951). *Gestalt therapy: Excitement and growth in the human personality*. Julian Press.

Sabar, S. (2000). Bereavement, grief and mourning: A Gestalt perspective. *Gestalt Review*, 4(2), 152–168.

Smith, E. (1985). A Gestalt therapist's perspective on grief. *Psychotherapy Patient*, 2(1), 65–78.

Vymětal, J. (2003). *Úvod do psychoterapie*. Grada Publishing.

Chapter 7

The Art of "Doing Nothing"

We can view a therapist's professional development as a process of the gradual release of attention capacity. It's like learning to drive a car. At first, there's an awful lot going on at once – our legs, hands, eyes, ears are working simultaneously. We need to be so aware of so much that it requires all our attention. After a few minutes of driving a car for the first time, we are sweaty and exhausted. In a few years, we will be doing all the same things while driving a car, but we will be able to calmly chat with a passenger, listen to music, even rest at the same time. We gradually need less and less attention to drive a car, and relaxed attention allows us to perceive and enjoy more and more aspects of what is happening.

Surviving on the Therapist's Chair

As nascent psychotherapists, we first learn to observe the client and understand what is happening with them. We learn to simultaneously separate our own processes and content, which distort our observation and understanding. And from our understanding we learn to create guidelines for what would be good to do and what would not. Assembling all this, we create a certain comprehensive idea of the therapeutic situation and what is needed next. For example, we see that the client is falling into a depressed mood and is exhausted. We understand that they need to save energy and reduce their expectations of themselves. Thus, we pose less challenging and more specific questions.

Learning in this way is crucial for us personally because it helps us survive in the therapist's position. The client does not really need us to be able to observe, understand and intervene well. Rather, it is what we need in order to cope with the new role in which we take on great responsibility and place great demands on ourselves.

At the beginning, we are gripped by anxiety and doubt. By learning, we help ourselves to survive in the role of a therapist. Later, this learning helps us settle into the therapist's role. And when we somehow learn to observe, understand and intervene, relief and knowledge will come: Ah, so this is psychotherapy! I can actually do this. After a few years of psychotherapeutic work with clients, we can say: Yes, I am a psychotherapist.

DOI: 10.4324/9781003500148-8

Learning the Craft

Once we have learned to "do" psychotherapy and are relieved that we can handle it from the position of a therapist, our attention capacity is freed up. We can then focus this attention on ourselves. On what happens with us in the presence of a client. We learn to observe ourselves, understand ourselves and direct our interventions accordingly. Our observation and understanding about the psychotherapy situation is thus enriched by information about the therapist. For example, we notice that we are uncomfortable when a client complains too much about how their depression is incapacitating. We explore this as a reflection on our own process as well as a co-created relational pattern.

After some time, we learn to quickly switch attention from the client to ourselves and back, observe both sides and understand what is happening between us and the client. We understand the craft, which suddenly moves easily by itself. Like driving a car as an experienced driver. Ah, so this is psychotherapy! Suddenly we don't have to think much about everything that is going on and what we are doing. This frees up our attention capacity. We calm down, quiet down. We are settled into the position of therapist and know that we fulfill this role well enough.

Feeling the Other

This is when we begin to really feel the other person as a unique being whose story has intersected with our story at this very moment, in this very place. We used to see the client and now we suddenly feel them. We have the capacity for this now because we no longer need to reassure ourselves that we understand what is happening and that we know what to do.

We no longer have to rescue ourselves by somehow intervening, by doing something. We stop helping the other as a means of running away from our anxious powerlessness. We now have the capacity to feel the uniqueness of the other, the uniqueness of ourselves, the uniqueness of each moment. To open up to the adventure of the moment. To open up to an encounter and its flow.

We have the capacity to work with ourselves, to transform how we are present, to transform our way of being. Sometimes, we can even, for example, sit freely in depressed powerlessness and hopelessness with the client. So this is psychotherapy! We allow ourselves to be aesthetically, via the senses, carried along by the current of subsequent moments. We lean into the inclination of the situation.[1]

As our capacity gradually frees up, we can perceive more of the infinitely rich whole of the situation in which we find ourselves with the client. At the same time, our anchoring in the position of therapist allows us not to cling to our understanding of what is happening. We are freer to create different versions of understanding depending on the perspective from which we choose to view the client and ourselves. More possibilities emerge for our meaningful interpretation of what we do in psychotherapy, as well as who we are and how we are in psychotherapy.

What the Self Sounds Like

The self can be perceived as a structure as well as a process. Both views have their merit and a therapist can use either to the benefit of the client. If we understand the self as a structure, it allows us to grasp psychological and relational processes. Then, for example, we can define mental content, such as intrapsychic polarities or subpersonalities, and the relationships between them, or different levels in the structure of the psyche and stages of development.

Viewing the self as a structure provides the therapist with reassurance through understanding and orientation. Such reassurance can be very functional, as it transfers from the therapist to the entire therapeutic situation and thus brings reassurance to the client. However, it is not without a flipside. It may be very tempting for the therapist to escape the chaos they experience by being exposed to the ever-changing and unique processes taking place in a psychotherapy situation. These processes are in essence as incomprehensible as the flow of a river. The risk is that the therapist will cease to stay attuned to this fluid reality and instead get stuck in the structuring theoretical concepts used for grasping this reality.

That is why the second concept of self is also important. The self as a process. This concept loosens our constructs and retunes us to seeing the incomprehensible changeability of reality, like listening to music. We can hold these two conceptions of self at the same time, as figure and ground, which continuously transform (Yontef, 1993) according to what is useful for the psychotherapeutic situation. Seeing the self as a structure brings us therapists comfort, seeing the self as a process brings us humility.

Here we focus on the self as a process and use the concept developed by Gestalt therapy. Emphasis on the self as a process is especially important for working with depression, because it is very difficult to perceive the flow of the process in a stiff and drained depressive atmosphere. That is why we need to focus on this process and become sensitive to the perception of even the slightest of movements.

Let us try to perceive the self as a river that flows, flows away, while still being present (Vázquez-Bandín, 2016). Self, a fluid process of being, is very difficult to capture in nouns; its flowing essence is better captured in verbs. Instead of self, we can use the term *selfing* (Parlett, 2005). Such a concept is also reflected in our thinking about psychopathology. Instead of labeling a person as depressed, we switch to a process concept and see the process of "depressing" in which the psychopathological field actualizes in a psychotherapeutic situation (Francesetti, 2012, 2015; Spagnuolo Lobb, 2013; Robine, 2011). Client and therapist thus "depress" together (Roubal, 2007, 2015; Francesetti & Roubal, 2013). If we see client and therapist as processes, as functions of the movements of the situation, then not only do they create depression together, but they themselves are formed by depression.

In order for a person to be able to experience contact with the surrounding world, they need to differentiate themselves from their surroundings.

From this point of view, the self is an emergent phenomenon (Philippson, 2001) of the present situation, a differentiation process in which the experience of the self is created moment by moment. Its creation begins with sensory perception, at which point there is not yet distinction between the subject and the world. Thus, prior to the emergence of the individual self, there is a bodily-experienced undefined situational self (Perls, Hefferline & Goodman, 1951; Robine, 2011). Only then does differentiation from the environment take place, but firstly just precognitively. We will now hone in on this bodily-experienced and precognitive, i.e. not actually describable in words and concepts, process.

Three Functions of the Self

The self as a process is uncapturable. But we can observe how this process takes shape. As if we were looking at a river to see where it turns, where it splashes, where it flows fast and where it calms down. One way to sensitize ourselves to the perception of these various movements is through the theoretical concept of *self functions*.[2] In order to understand them, it is important to emphasize that these functions do not belong to an individual, they do not describe their characteristics, but they continuously evolve from the current situation. They are functions of the field dynamics.

We can imagine the function of the self through the metaphor of music. If we listen to the self as a melody, we can try to recognize what instruments are playing this melody. We may hear three – say a flute, a piano and a bass. Together, these three instruments seem to create the melody of the self. At the same time, it is very practical for psychotherapists to learn to listen to each of them separately, because in certain situations in psychotherapy, one of the instruments may need our special care.

Instrument one: what we do (*ego function of the self*). What the client does in a given situation, what the therapist does, what we do together. It is an executive function by which we creatively enter the world around us, leave our mark on it and give it shape. Perhaps we could call it *shaping*. What we do – here, we mean this in terms of behavior and actively performed activity. So not only our actions, but also our understanding. How we use our thinking to creatively grasp what is happening.

Instrument two: who we are (*personality function of the self*), who we become for each other. How client and therapist relate to each other. And what stories lead them to their encounter. It is a function describing interpersonal adjustment. Perhaps we could call it *relating*. Who we become for each other in the flow of the situation. And how who we are to each other, as two co-created processes, gets transformed in the flow of the situation here and now.

Instrument three: how we are (*id function of the self*). How client and therapist, as two beings of flesh and blood, dwell together in this world. It is the way of our embodied being in the present situation. This function of the self could perhaps be called *"bellying."* Needs arising from the situation emerge through the body and the senses. This function describes the bodily and synesthetic experiences of being in the present (i.e. preverbal processes), and therefore it is difficult to capture in words.

What we do, who we are, how we are. Flute, piano, bass. As therapists, we listen to how loud each instrument plays. We can then support the one that is quiet or faint. For example, when physical involvement (*id function*) is missing, we can invite it to be more present. We can ask about how the client feels in their body. But we can draw it out even through ourselves. We can notice our body and listen to how it is doing in a given situation. Perhaps our body, which is a sensitive receptor, is expressing some needs in the current situation.

Or perhaps the flute sounds very loud and has long been playing so loudly that the other instruments cannot be heard. Psychotherapy is saturated with action, finding solutions to problems, reasoning about what would be good to do. And a therapist can instead listen more closely to the piano. Invite it to play louder: who we are for each other at this moment (*personality function*) when we look for a solution in this way. It may turn out that we are fixed in some relational pattern, perhaps as victim and savior. Then maybe one needs to play the piano more creatively, step out of the position of savior and try to be a guide. Mutual relating will change and so will the victim.

Here, the volume of the instruments is a metaphor for the focus of attention. Where the therapist directs attention and how much they focus in that direction. That is, how much weight they assign to each self function at a given moment. Let us now look at one illustrative case study fragment:

First session. Victor: "I'm depressed."

Therapist: (Right from the start I perceive an implicit claim on me, as if the whole sentence was actually: "I'm depressed and you do something about it." I don't want to rise to it, instead I want to divide the responsibility for the change, share it. I need to pull him in more.)

"Hmm... And would you tell me more about it? What's it like?"

"Well, I just feel sick..."

(I hear: "I don't want to talk about it, just cure me of it." Okay, I'll try a roundabout way.)

"Can you sleep at night?"

"Well, that's just it, I'm completely worn out. I wake up at three and stare into the dark."

(It seems easier for him to answer specific questions that are a bit peripheral to the main suffering.)

"How long has it been like this?"

"I don't even know, an awfully long time."

"And do you take any medication to help?"

"Yeah, antidepressants, third ones already, no use... I just fall asleep a bit better with them, but then I'm wiped all day. It's just useless..."

(I hear: "I'm useless." As if I could feel the darkness, the dark despair in my stomach. He opens the door for me to take a peek at how he feels through my own experience. I can only get to him like this, indirectly.)

"Hmm..."

"So they sent me here to you."

(Again, there's this implicit expectation that I'll do something about it, but now it's more like a very cautious hope. I no longer feel pressured to do something about it. More like, "Please, could you do something about me? I can't anymore.")

"Yeah, I see you're really not feeling well."

"Yeah..."

(He looks at me as if for the first time he was giving a chance to the possibility of me hearing him. I don't want to scare it off, I'd better still go around.)

"Do you manage to go to work?"

"Well that's the thing, I can't anymore... I tried to push through for a long time, but my strength has run out. I've been on sick leave for over two months now, and it's just getting worse and worse."

(Careful now, little by little the possibility that he will start sharing his suffering with me is starting to open. But I mustn't scare it off by starting to comfort him or giving him optimism.)

"You have no strength. Probably no joy in life, either?'

"No, I really don't have that. I'm at rock bottom. Worn out, sleep deprived, I can't manage anything, my wife doesn't give a damn about me, the children too..."

(I see how he revives a little, paradoxically. His shoulders relax, he looks at me again, a little inquisitively, who am I?)

"You're at rock bottom..." (I show a downward motion with my hands, a downward wave, stopping at the lowest point.) "That's how you sank to the bottom, yes?"

"Yeah, exactly."

"Did something happen at the beginning?" (I point to the beginning of the falling of the wave.)

"I don't know, I guess not. Everything normal, over and over again, work, family. Just a normal guy in his forties."

"Do you think the forties have something to do with it?"

"I don't know. But I'm already a write-off."

(So a moment ago I thought that I could hold on to the forties, that it might be some kind of a transformational mid-life crisis. I would be relieved if that were the case, I would know where to direct the therapy. But he doesn't respond to that. It makes sense. If I held on to the expectation of how therapy might work, I'd be relieved. I'd feel better and due to that I'd leave him experientially. But he needs me to stick with him on the dark side, into the murkiness and the uncertainty. All right then.)

"As if you have nothing in front of you..."

"Exactly."

Nothing has happened in therapy yet. Victor is still depressed and I learned some rather vague information. We did not agree on what would happen in therapy. On an explicit level, nothing new has occurred, nothing that would promise change. Yet a lot is happening under the surface, implicitly. The relationship is getting transformed: from a lonely pushing away to a hint of an alliance in the dark. And the atmosphere is transforming too: from tense, cold despair to painful sorrow.

Let us now use the theory of the three functions of the self to understand what is happening at different levels in this therapeutic situation. We hear the flute the most in the foreground. What we do (*ego function*). The therapist tries doing something, asks what the client is doing with his depression. The client in turn wants the therapist to do something. It seems to go in a loop at this level of doing. The client informs: I've already done everything possible, nothing works, now you do something with me. And the therapist: until you do something, I won't do anything with you. It loops around and around.

But big things happen implicitly at the level of relating (*personality function*). Nothing is clear there, only movement. As if the piano was improvising and looking for a melody. In the beginning, Victor is the one asking the therapist to fix him. He doesn't beg, he asks. Angrily because he resents the powerless position this puts him in. And the therapist does not want to be the repairman of the passively dysfunctional Victor. He does not respond to the aggressive tone in which Victor asks for fixing. Instead, he diverts attention elsewhere, explores. The therapist becomes an explorer instead of a repairman. And who does Victor become? It is not yet clear, but in any case, the possibility opens up to step out of the position of the dysfunctional and angry helpless one. Perhaps toward the end of the case study fragment, Victor becomes a little bit like a little boy who fell, scraped his knee and tries not to cry. And who does the therapist become? The piano melody seems to start resonating.

What about the bass? Describing the physical way of being (*id-function*) is always the most difficult. We often do not even notice the bass. We only notice when it stops playing. The bass is heard in the fact that together, Victor and the therapist remain physically, as two beings, in the same room. And that together they are slowly settling down. It is as if at the start Victor was present in a weary way: *if it isn't good for me here, I'll run away*. And the therapist was present in an exhausted way: *someone wants something from me again, I'd rather be somewhere else*. But this slowly changes. Imperceptibly, the bass begins to consolidate a rhythm, creating a safe background for collaboration. Toward the end of the illustrative case study fragment, Victor sits in the room in this manner: *here I can allow myself to feel sick*. And the therapist: *I'm sitting here, in a fragile moment, moved. I want to give this a chance by staying here with Victor. I'll try to sit out hope.*

The Helpless Therapist

We now return to a concept from the beginning of this chapter – that of the therapist's development. We find that, along with professional development, a key therapeutic competence can develop: coping with one's own powerlessness. We will probably be unable to stay out of the way without this competence. So let us study powerlessness for a moment through the lenses of the already familiar three perspectives, centered either on a person, on a relationship, or on a field.

Elisabeth is an elderly lady who feels so lonely and longs for human touch so much that her "skin hurts." She fell into depression during the pandemic lockdown. In particular, she suffered from the fact that no one, out in the world, was waiting for her after the end of the lockdown. She turns to me with a stiff, expressionless face. Her look screams, "This is unbearable. Help me!" I feel helpless. What should I do? What can I do? I'm sorry, I can't help you... powerlessness.

Powerlessness (and also its companion hopelessness) sits with us in the psychotherapy office and fill us with every breath. This, very naturally, awakens self-preservation impulses in us through our bodies, which lead us to activity. An active approach aimed at change allows us to emerge from unbearable powerlessness face to face with a suffering person for whom we are the only hope. At the same time, we polarize ourselves against the client, leaving them unaccepted in their suffering. By doing so, we only further strengthen the powerlessness of the situation. We thus need to start with ourselves, with our experience of powerlessness.

How can we manage our own powerlessness? This again depends on the point of view, on the perspective from which we view psychothcrapcutic processes. As psychotherapists, we work in three parallel modes: (1) we do something, (2) we relate in some way, and (3) we are in some way essentially, bodily present. All three of these modes are useful, and at different stages of the therapeutic process each one of them comes to the foreground and the others recede into the background. Each of them is based on a different theoretical perspective from which we understand how we as therapists can manage our own powerlessness.

From a mono-personal perspective, we as therapists focus on raising awareness within a uniquely supportive therapeutic relationship (accepting the person and challenging their fixed patterns) and aim to increase the capacity for new creative adaptation. As already mentioned, we work like a gardener who waters, digs around, but does not pull on the flower to make it grow faster.

We work with our own experience of *powerlessness* by noticing it, labeling it and processing it in supervision. We often find that it is about the high demands we make on ourselves in therapy (*I should help the client*) and on the client (*they should change faster*). Eventually, when the client is ready for it, we can put a name to our own powerlessness directly in front of them. We can then use this either as a self-revealing confession in order to humanize the expert, or as feedback on how other people may feel around the client. Basically, we help the client be able to help themselves. And by our helping, we help ourselves not to feel helpless.

We also, parallel to what we do in psychotherapy, relate to a client in a certain way. From the bi-personal, we as therapists focus on the relational experience co-created in the therapeutic relationship by the client and us. What matters is who we become for each other, what "old dance" we dance together and what "new steps" emerge. The therapist's job is to enable a new relational experience by relating to the client openly, genuinely as a person, so that the client feels accepted as they are.

We then perceive our own powerlessness as an assessment of our share in the co-created relational pattern and of the dynamics of the psychotherapeutic relationship. We can illustrate such a dynamic on the example of a therapist's experience translated into inner dialogue:

> *I feel helpless with you. Why are you doing this to me?! Why don't you cooperate a little more? You pretend to be the victim of the situation: others are to blame for everything. You are passive aggressive. To me too. And I'm powerless, it's so uncomfortable. And you are to blame!*

It is the frequent victim-persecutor constellation with the positions reversed. The therapist protects themselves against their own experience of powerlessness by aggressively rejecting the client.

As therapists, we are trained to be sensitive to such experiences, to notice them before they destroy the slowly and patiently woven web of a safe therapeutic relationship. We note our contribution to the repetitive co-created relational pattern, we realize how we step on the client's toes with our learned old dance. And we then consciously change our contribution to the co-created pattern. Again, let's hear this as internal dialogue:

> *I feel so helpless with you! It's very uncomfortable. Well, I'm not here to be comfortable. This profession is my choice, working with you is my decision. I feel helpless because I would like to help you change the terribly unsatisfying life you are living. But unfortunately it is not within my power. But I can provide you with a safe place here in therapy and offer you a chance for change that starts with yourself. That's my offer, that's what I'm sitting here with, not just powerlessness.*

We step out of the repetitive relationship pattern, as if inviting the client in for a visit. We invite them in from the dangerous and unsatisfying world to visit the safe acceptance of a therapeutic relationship. This also helps us to escape the feeling of powerlessness.

In psychotherapy, we not only do something and relate to the client in some way, but we also simultaneously function in another mode: the mode of being. We are present. Bodily, essentially. From the field theory perspective, we as therapists focus on the processes by which the current situation organizes. We perceive the field structuring movements. And we also tune in to the intentionality of the situation, i.e. to processes that are not yet happening, but are present in the form of a possibility. In other words, that which can happen given sufficient support.

It is as if we are in the water with the client, carried by a current that exceeds us. Our task is to let ourselves be carried by the flow of the situation, while concurrently transforming the way of our own being in the situation, so as to make room for the natural flow of presence. We then perceive, mainly corporeally, our own *powerlessness* as a report on the process of which we are a function at this moment. On the current that swept us. On the power of powerlessness that shapes client and therapist.

Our powerlessness makes us feel the client's powerlessness. Our powerlessness creates a bridge to the client, but a strange, underwater bridge, present implicitly through our embodied being in the situation. The connection between us is that we stay sitting together, that our bodies stay seated together even when we are helpless.

We sit together in powerlessness, and by doing so, we rid the powerlessness of loneliness. Here, we do not invite the client for a visit. Instead, by delving into our own powerlessness, we leave our cozy safety and go visit the client. We experience firsthand what it is like to be them. How helpless it is. We remain in our own bodily experienced powerlessness – and wait to see what happens. We surrender to the flow of the situation.

A path will appear, it will emerge from the process and the current of powerlessness will carry us to where the path begins. But we have to make room for it. The path has not yet appeared because it lacked space. We must not get in the way of change by overtaking its place with our good intentions and efforts to help. It is about not filling the space for change with yourself, but making room for hope instead. To be quiet enough to notice what wants to be heard. To be slow enough not to miss what is not yet in being.

By being truly present in a helpless way and not trying to change this state of being, we provide support to the field processes that are therefore able to emerge. We can then welcome the experience of powerlessness as an invitation, as an open door for what is missing in the given situation and what longs to happen.

We make room for it by not helping. We try to gather the courage to "do nothing" in the face of a suffering person. For ourselves, for our body sitting here, we can repeat a mantra in our minds: *I don't want to change you. I want to be in it with you. I want to feel powerlessness with you and be carried by it.* Again and again we resist the impulses that tempt us to flee from the experience of powerlessness.

This powerlessness is a chance to be present without one's own power. It is an opportunity to give up our own power and let forces that exceed us be the help. It is not so important what we do, but how we are with the client. We remain in the powerlessness, we give up, and at the same time we feel hope. Perhaps we could go even further and let ourselves be carried by hopelessness as well. Instead of swimming to the solid shore of hope, we could share hopelessness with the client, even use that shared hopelessness to strengthen the bridge between us. After all, the client feels hopeless and I connect with them through it; we share powerlessness and hopelessness.

The process of change in the psychotherapy of depression can be seen as transforming an *abyss* into a *fertile void*.[3] If we understand the client's suffering in depression as a desire for another, we can understand our own sense of powerlessness as evidence that we perceive this desire. Proof that we do not leave the client alone in it. In the course of psychotherapy, interpersonal emptiness is transformed into an experience of shared emptiness, which ceases to be empty thanks to being shared.

As therapists, we enable such a transformation by the way we are present in a depressive situation: by putting ourselves at risk and exposing ourselves to the archaic fear of the depressive emptiness without protecting ourselves with therapeutic approach and interventions. Yet, in closing this chapter, it is important to say that this does not mean sitting with the client and not doing anything. Especially with a depressed client, it is important for the therapist to keep an active and structured approach, limiting long empty moments during which the client could sink even more into hopeless abandonment. So of course we do something. But at the same time, we do not expect anything from it. We surrender to powerlessness and remain curious about where it will take us. We are present this way. And from this position we do something.

Notes

1   This frees up our attention capacity. What we do with it, I don't know, I didn't get further than this. I have a small suspicion that in the next stage we will stop doing psychotherapy altogether, but what do I know?

2   This concept is a creative elaboration of the original inspiration from psychoanalysis, which the founders of Gestalt therapy converted into a process and relational concept (Perls, Hefferline & Goodman, 1951) and which was developed especially by I. Fromm (Spagnuolo Lobb, 2005).

3   In the theory of Gestalt therapy, the term fertile void describes bodily experienced notknowing in the phase preceding contact (fore-contact). In this state, it is possible to experience how the forthcoming contact is already shaping us (Jacobs, 2020). Experiencing this pre-contact enabling differentiation phase (pre-difference) (Perls, 1969) is key to the creative process of change and the reorganization of the psychopathological field (Amendt-Lyon, 2020).

Bibliography

Amendt-Lyon, N. (2020). How can a void be fertile? Implications of Friedlaender's creative indifference for Gestalt therapy theory and practice. *Gestalt Review*, 24(2), 142–162.

Di Lampedusa, G. T. (1960). *The Leopard*. Pantheon.

Francesetti, G. (2012). Pain and beauty: From psychopathology to the aesthetics of contact. *British Gestalt Journal*, 21(2), 4–18.

Francesetti, G. (2015). From individual symptoms to psychopathological fields: Towards a field perspective on clinical human suffering. *British Gestalt Journal*, 24(1), 5–19.

Francesetti, G., Roubal, J. (2013) Gestalt therapy approach to depressive experiences. In Francesetti, G., Gecele, M., Roubal, J. (Eds.), *Gestalt therapy in clinical practice: From psychopathology to the aesthetics of contact*. Franco Angeli, 433–494.

Jacobs, L. (2020). Engaged surrender: The polarity of dialogue in Gestalt therapy. *Gestalt Review*, 24(2), 163–177.

Parlett, M. (2005). Contemporary Gestalt therapy: Field theory. In Woldt, A. L., Toman, M. (Eds.), *Gestalt therapy: History, theory, and practice*. Sage Publications, 41–64.

Perls, F. (1969). *Ego, hunger and aggression: The beginnings of Gestalt therapy*. Random House.

Perls, F., Hefferline, R. F., Goodman, P. (1951). *Gestalt therapy: Excitement and growth in the human personality*. Julian Press.

Philippson, P. (2001). *Self in relation*. Karnac Books.

Robine, J. M. (2011). *On the occasion of an other.* Gestalt Journal Press.

Roubal, J. (2007). Depression – a Gestalt theoretical perspective. *British Gestalt Journal*, 16(1), 35–43.

Roubal, J. (2015). Depressing together: Therapist's experience in a therapy situation with a depressed client. In Francesetti, G. (Ed.), *Absence is the bridge between us (Gestalt Therapy Book Series, 20)*. Intituto di Gestalt HCC, 205–224.

Spagnuolo Lobb, M. (2005). Classical Gestalt therapy theory. In Woldt, A. L., Toman, M. (Eds.), *Gestalt therapy. history, theory, and practice*. Sage Publications, 21–39.

Spagnuolo Lobb, M. (2013). *The now-for-next in psychotherapy: Gestalt therapy recounted in post-modern society*. FrancoAngeli.

Vázquez-Bandin, C. (2016) *In Self: A polyphony of Gestalt therapists*. Edited by J.-M. Robine. L'Exprimeire.

Yontef, G. (1993). *Awareness, dialogue and process: Essays on Gestalt therapy.* Gestalt Journal Press.

Chapter 8

Surrendering to Hope

Choosing not to help and thus not to escape from the heavy powerlessness is a very active, demanding process. It is the art of "doing nothing." As if what we do and who we are were not as important for the moment.[1] We risk ourselves and let ourselves be shaped by the field movements. We become part of the client's suffering, which actualizes in the present situation.

Here we find ourselves in a fundamental dilemma (Francesetti & Roubal, 2020): how can we participate in a psychopathological process and at the same time not reinforce it? How can we be accepting of the clinical situation, of the client and their symptoms, and at the same time not give up on change, and still hold on to hope? The field theory perspective allows us to step out of this dilemma in a way that is brilliantly described by the concept of *the paradoxical theory of change*:[2] "Change occurs when one becomes what he is, not when he tries to become what he is not" (Beisser, 1970, p. 88). How does this translate into therapeutic work? We learn to trust that the therapeutic situation will change if we fully accept it as it is. That it will change if we do not try to change it. The paradoxical theory of change helps us trust that the process of change happens on its own, often in unexpected and unpredictable ways. It gives us confidence that when we step into a void, we land on solid ground and that this landing will give meaning to our step (Perls, Hefferline & Goodman, 1951, p. 123).

When we look at the psychotherapy process from a field theory perspective, it leads us to be humbled before the healing processes and before the field movements that transcend both the individual and the therapeutic relationship (Roubal & Francesetti, 2022). As therapists, we can support change by accepting the therapeutic situation, by really settling down into it. We can start, for example, by becoming fully aware of our presence in contact with another:

Michael was fired from his job eight months ago, and he has been falling into depression ever since. He has nothing to live for, nothing makes him happy, he has no strength for anything. I'm sitting across from him and I'm thinking to myself, "Yeah, it's damn hard! It's hard for me too. I'm tired, nothing works, it's like talking into a black hole. But maybe just sitting here with him has its worth. But I don't want to be sitting here. I want to go outside, walk among the trees, be

DOI: 10.4324/9781003500148-9

at home with my family, be with myself, I don't want to sit here. My body doesn't want to sit here, my ass actually hurts sitting on this chair, that's how much it doesn't want to be here."

At this moment, the real, existential choice occurs. I'm here, and I don't want to be. But I am, there's nothing I can do about it. It's an ethical question, my responsibility. I am responsible to the reality as it is, that I am sitting here. Since I'm already sitting here, since my body is already sitting here, I'm supposed to be here too. With my physical presence, I promise to be here, I assume the obligation to be here. I choose to be consciously in this moment here in this room with this person. It's a fundamental decision to say to yourself: "Yes, I'm dedicating this moment of my life to meeting this person here, to really being with him." After all, what other choice is there, I'm here anyway. I don't really have a choice. My choice lies in honestly accepting my responsibility. "Since I'm here, I'll be here. I see you in front of me, I feel myself here with you. I am here with you."

Together with the client, we let ourselves be carried by the current that shapes our meeting. In the case of depression, it is rather a very slow-moving, swampy current. We are settled in the present situation. We see it without delusions and we accept it. We do not shrug off the burden, we do not comfort the sadness; instead, we respectfully stay present with what is. We float through the swamp, drifting along with the slow muddy current:

I am sitting on a chair, in a room, with Michael. This is simply how reality looks, which I therefore accept and from which I can push off. I see Michael in front of me. I see him lowering his head, dandruff falling from his unwashed hair onto his shirt. I hear his quiet, monotone voice. Fragments of what he says reach me: ... "I don't know how... It's been too much... she says... it probably won't be possible..." As if his words were too frail to reach me. As if they withered on the way from his chair to mine. This too seems to be the reality of our situation. The atmosphere is so heavy that the words fall to the ground before reaching the other. What can be done in such an atmosphere? I don't know. I try to breathe in the atmosphere. It actually works pretty well, I'm actually breathing well. And at that moment I hear: ... "because I simply couldn't keep up with the youngsters anymore..." As if I inhaled those words. It seems that it is necessary not only to listen to the words, but to directly inhale them. Quite a strange image. I exhale the answer:

"And you want to keep up with them, the youngsters?"

"Well, they're just in a different place... different age... I'm already..."

Words don't have the power to fly over again. But I noticed that he responded to my question by raising his eyes and looking at me. As if the surface of the oppressive atmosphere rippled a little. So I try again, see what it does.

"You know, I'm genuinely curious whether you want to keep up with the youngsters. I imagine it like you riding a bike with them. Do you want to go as fast as them?"

"I won't be able to anyway. I don't have the strength for it. I wouldn't even be able to stay on a bike now. Since I don't sleep, so... legs..."

Of course, it's not that easy. Again, an oppressive atmosphere washes over us both, separates us from each other. I had this nice idea that maybe he could figure out his own pace in life. And that he could then leave the faster pace to the younger generations and find a pace that would be good for him in his current life situation. The intervention itself might have been all right, but it didn't help bring about change, because I was saying it with my own internal motivation: I would like to push the situation in this direction. I did not remain free and open in order to curiously welcome whatever comes. Instead, I preferred the situation to move in a certain direction. By trying to help Michael with a good idea, I only further strengthened both his powerless position as well as the oppressive atmosphere through which we could not reach one another. I myself was not accepting the situation and I unreservedly tried to jump out of the flow of the swampy current.

It is essential for therapeutic work that we focus not on what we do, but from where we do it. How present we are in the moment when we undertake a certain intervention. It is key for our intervention, whatever it may be, to come from a place that is free from expectations. We need to wait for a state in which we freely follow our curiosity and do not expect results. Then our keen interest will guide us through the swamp of depression. It is as if our keen interest shows us where the situation wants to move next. As if it indicates a current that can be set in motion thanks to our free presence.

Michael utters weak words into the oppressive atmosphere: "I won't be able to anyway. I don't have the strength for it. I wouldn't even be able to stay on a bike now. Since I don't sleep, so... legs..."

I sink deeper into the chair, falling asleep. Not yet really, but I'm not far from it. But I already know that it helps to breathe. Inhale as I listen. Exhale to answer:

"Hmm... you're not sleeping... And what do you do when you're not sleeping?"

"What? I just lie there, turn over."

"Are you thinking about something?"

"Yeah, I guess so... About everything that I... screwed up..."

"And what did you screw up?"

"Everything... Work, family, marriage, life... everything."

That is strange. The words seem to suddenly have the power to fly all the way to me. I hear Michael clearly, I see him, he is looking at me.

"I see. I'm trying to understand what you're saying. Could it be that you had some vision of what your life would be like and it turned out differently?"

"Yeah, I guess, something like that... it turned out bad..."

"It didn't work out as you imagined?"

"No, it didn't. But why the hell not?"

The words are very clear now, even sharp. I can hear Michael without a problem, the change is obvious. However, what that means and what I should do is not very clear to me.

"Would you mind telling me about it, please? Why the hell it didn't work out? How do you make sense of it?"

"Well, I guess I'm not that cool..."

"... as you thought..."

"...as my dad or brother."

"Are you different?"

"I'm a wuss."

"A wuss?"

"Yeah, a wuss."

"I don't understand. What do you mean?"

"I don't really understand it either, but that's what they always told me at home. Michael, don't be a wuss."

"And why not?"

And here something happens. I see revival in Michael's eyes. As if he was starting to feel me. As if he felt a living person next to him. He looks at me, maybe the corner of his mouth even twitches with a hint of a smile. So I try staying the course:

"Could we linger on this for a second? Why shouldn't you be a wuss?"

"Well, I'd say it doesn't matter anymore. I screwed everything up, so now I can be a wuss."

"Hmm, yeah, that makes sense."

I try a tiny, slightly sly smile. Michael's mask moves, his expression is different than before. Somewhat sullen, but at the same time perhaps also somewhat covert. The atmosphere is still oppressive, but it's almost as if it weren't quite the same everywhere. As if there were vents in it to crawl through. This is how I imagine change.

The aesthetically perceived transformation of the atmosphere is at that moment the change that appeared by itself. There was an unexpected change in the atmosphere of our meeting: it is still oppressive, but possibilities of connection have opened up through sullenness and covertness. It's a very small change, but I think a significant one. As if the switch has flipped on how the process will continue to unfold. As if it's offering directions to somewhere Michael isn't used to going in conversations with others.

Also, new interesting topics have emerged – for example, the demands on oneself and the related relationship with father and brother – these alone will not be too difficult to work with. But if we were to work with them in the original oppressive atmosphere in which we couldn't reach each other, it probably wouldn't lead to change. We would discuss his demands and his relationships in the family and... it would still be the same experientially. Here, however, from the last moments of our conversation, it seems hopeful that our further work could already take place in a slightly experientially altered atmosphere. The background of our meeting is changing, from which new and unexpected figures may emerge.

As therapists, we do not make change, we just open the door for it. We thus allow for change that we cannot arrange, or even foresee. If we want to be instrumental to change, we must not try to arrange or manage it. It is enough for us to be present with what is. Radically speaking: it is not important what we do, but how we are. It could also be said that whatever intervention we actively attempt, we do not actually expect any results. Intervention is important especially to reassure ourselves. To quiet down enough to be able to hear the silent call of the as-yet-absent natural flow of the situation, which longs to be freed from the prison of the psychopathological field organization. Then it is our task not to stand in the way of this incipient movement. To make room, by our way of being, for this movement to find its way through the unique conditions of the situation here and now.

How Might the Paradoxical Theory of Change Work

In order to flow freely like this with the current of change that is awakened by our flowing, we need the buttress of our accumulated experience – both personal and professional, both our own and shared. We need something to lean on. If we lack such support, we will probably experience restlessness and anxiety in a demanding clinical situation. We will not be sound in ourselves, in who we are in a given situation (*personality function*), and therefore it will probably be difficult for us to let go of our position. It will be hard to lose ourselves and let ourselves be carried away by what comes. Our own anxiety will likely force us to take care of ourselves and sideline the client for the moment. Our interventions to try to help the client will actually serve to alleviate our anxiety and strengthen our own position, so that we do not feel powerless in front of the suffering client.

This is how we become the one who is pulling the client out of depression. This simply defined, meaningful position brings a sense of relief. At the same time, however, we reduce the possibilities of the situation – the only options become either to pull out of depression or slide back into it – and thus close the door on other, unpredictable possibilities for change. It is the same as what happens to the client in other relationships. They don't need therapy for that.

We can therefore understand our anxiety in the therapist's position as a message to ourselves. As a signal that we do not have enough supportive ground under our feet to be able to tolerate the uncertainty while waiting for change, which may appear, but in its own time and in some unpredictable form.

You could say that when we try to help our clients, we reduce the situation's potential. We limit the options for change to what we believe would be good for the clients. Just with this helper mindset of ours, we ourselves become part of the psychopathological field organization, further strengthening it. Our efforts to help thus stand in the way of natural healing processes that try to free themselves from the psychopathological field organization.

If we want to encourage change, we need to not get in the way by helping. We need to be present without direction and expectation, to be able to let go of our good intentions. To not chase after what is not, but surrender to what already is.

To the hope present in the situation itself. It is a hope that manifests as a result of the fact that we are sitting here together with the client. If we manage to be present in this manner, we stop putting ourselves in the way and thereby free the field dynamic, regardless of whatever concrete form it then takes.

Not getting in the way of change with our efforts to help does not mean we stand completely aside as therapists. On the contrary, we are immersed in the flow of the situation, we let ourselves be carried by it. By not trying to induce change, we make room for change to transpire. We can repeat a mantra to ourselves when facing a depressed client: *I'm not here to help you. I just want to be here with you.* This shifts us away from performance expectations of ourselves and of the client and instead brings to the foreground how we are present (*id function*). We emphasize the critical importance of how we are present.

The more we manage to anchor ourselves within, the more we will be able to free ourselves from the task of arranging change. From such a free position we can then be available to the field movements. We can follow these movements, experience them bodily, but not identify with them. We perceive them with our senses, experience them with emotions and let them flow through us. We truly experience them, and at the same time we do not appropriate them. As if what we are really experiencing is at the same time not quite so personal. Instead of it being our own experience – "I'm happy, I'm scared" – it is more like visiting the experience – "It made me happy, I got scared." We can trust how our feelings emerge in a clinical situation and take them absolutely seriously. Because whatever the emotions, they always belong to the situation, they are a function of it. And we remain curious and free toward them.

Such interested and anchored freedom is important, because it allows us not to hold onto who we are in the moment. It allows us to risk ourselves and, through our body, to let ourselves be carried in the direction of the *intentionality of the situation.* In the direction of a nascent movement that invites us to participate in change. We are able to sense the door that is waiting as a still unfulfilled possibility. It can then materialize and crack open thanks to our free acceptance of whatever arises in the given situation. We allow ourselves to be moved by the field movements at the level of undifferentiated experience waiting to materialize. Then perhaps this new experience, which until now was only present as a possibility, might get a chance to become a reality.

Free Curiosity

The approach described above guides us in a paradoxical way. When we sit with a client and feel the urgency to do something, it is the right time to wait and "do nothing." That means holding off on our outwardly directed activity and instead focusing on ourselves. We do not abandon the client experientially, we just let them recede into the background for the given moment and feel ourselves in the foreground. The feeling of urgency informs us that we are not anchored in ourselves at the moment. That we are inclining toward our good intentions. That we are not sufficiently freely and impartially balanced.

At this point, we probably need to make some time to support ourselves. We anchor ourselves thanks to our body, our breath and our senses. We can also hold on to a theoretical third party (Francesetti, Gecele & Roubal, 2013) and try to understand the situation. Sometimes we experience an urgency that persists even between sessions. In such cases, we can get support via supervision or by turning to literature describing what drives us to activity (for example, the client's suicidal thoughts or severe psychosomatic manifestations). With all this, we build a supportive environment that enables us to not act toward the client out of our anxiety. So when we feel an urgency to do something in psychotherapy, we can again understand it as a message to ourselves. As another signal that it is necessary to attend to our own needs first.

Thanks to support, *anxiety* transforms to *excitement*. As therapists, we need the anxiety and sense of urgency we feel in a clinical situation to transform into excited curiosity. We need the freedom that such an inner transformation brings. So if we feel tension, urgency, or other limiting feelings, we must turn to ourselves first and support ourselves. Then we can lean on ourselves and freely let ourselves be carried by the psychopathological field movements. We do not need to intervene. We can, and we don't need to. And that, paradoxically, is exactly the right time to intervene. Whatever action we take from such a free position has a chance to resound as an answer to the call of the situation.

Often our self-support work is not conscious, it is not as if we say to ourselves, "Now I will transform my tension into curiosity." It happens rather intuitively and therefore much faster than cognitive understanding. The transformation of our experience takes place on a preverbal, physical level. The way we are bodily present with the client changes (*id function*). We let our physically perceived needs for anchoring, calming and strengthening come to the foreground.

Paradoxically then, our interventions will not be aimed at the client, but at ourselves. When we feel tension in our body, when urgency presses our shoulders together and our whole body forward toward the client, we must take a moment before intervening. First, we need to support ourselves bodily. For example, we can sit up straight or lean against the back of the chair, release the tension in our muscles, and start breathing freely. This may well be enough to turn our anxiety into curious excitement. Such small interventions directed at our own body can take place many times in a session, often without conscious decision.

So we encourage our physical being in a situation (*id function*) to come to the foreground. This changes who we are in a given situation (*personality function*). We can then lean on ourselves and we can risk ourselves. We can risk stepping out of the safe and constraining position of one who is responsible for change and instead make ourselves available and be in service of what arises. We offer ourselves to be used by the change in order for it to happen. This is how who we are in a given situation with the client transforms: from one who is responsible for change, we become one who is available. Only then can we do something (*ego function*), because only then will our action be freed from expectations. Only then will it be a good time to direct attention back to the client and intervene.

Internal Work as a Speed Bump

From a practical point of view, it is essential to focus on the space between the moment in which we receive a certain impulse from a client and the moment in which we respond. We need to stretch this interval to make room for an in-between step, a moment for ourselves. If we were to intervene immediately, we would likely be trying to produce change before all the elements needed for holistic transformation had the chance to emerge. In doing so, we would only be repeating and reinforcing the psychopathological process of field organization, because we would be attempting to change it and we would not be accepting the situation in its entirety, as it is.

It is thus about briefly focusing on ourselves before responding to the client. We can learn to add this intermediate step and practice it so that it becomes a natural part of our psychotherapeutic work. So that it becomes part of our competence to work "in a field way." In principle, this is nothing revolutionary. When we look at how very experienced psychotherapists work, they do not seem to be doing anything special. They don't seem to have found a magical formula thanks to their wealth of experience. But we can observe that they are somewhat strangely slowed down. As if their reactions to clients were lagging.

Yes, they are slowed down, and what acts as a speed bump here is the in-between step that has become a natural part of their work over the years. The accumulated wisdom of their longtime work with clients teaches them the importance of waiting a moment before acting. And using this space to "do nothing." A moment of "doing nothing" before doing something. They know to create time for themselves when talking to the other, for a friendly dwelling with themselves. Every word, smile or sigh then becomes a powerful intervention because it comes from a free and anchored position. It responds to field callings and expects nothing.

Yet we as therapists are by no means passive in this receiving position. We just do not try to make change happen. We are talking about change as a holistic transformation that goes beyond our limited horizon. Such change cannot be made, much like you cannot make happiness. We prepare the ground for change, prepare a place for it, open the door to it by "doing nothing." "Doing nothing" is a very active process. We feel this, for example, because of how tired we are after such work. It is a specific tiredness, different from the drained tiredness that ensues when we try to help the client. Instead, this is a fulfilled tiredness, like the tiredness of a traveler who walks untrodden paths.

When "doing nothing," we are actually constantly letting go of our instinctive impulses to do something and thereby to react to the psychopathological forces organizing the present situation. We actively dissolve our tendencies to change the current situation. We open ourselves to whatever happens. In this way we welcome what is missing. What longs to become present, but has not yet had the space to do so. Therapy is thus encountering what is missing. Giving a voice to what wants to be heard. Then the present situation sets off in a new direction and becomes more whole.

We do not try for change, and in the meantime (as a result), change is already happening. The mycelium has changed, and whatever now grows out of it will be the change. So we do not try to change the depression, the visible part. We work with the background from which the clinical symptoms originally emerged as a figure. Through our embodied being, we create space for the possible transformation of the depressive situation's mycelium. This transformed mycelium then allows for other mushrooms to grow.

It is important to reiterate that this book is not a normative prescription of what the therapist should do. A whole variety of therapeutic interventions are possible. It depends on the personality of the therapist, the therapeutic relationship, the stage of therapy and the psychotherapeutic approach. Here, instead, we focus on the place from where the therapist is intervening. How they need to adjust their position first. How they retune themselves before doing something.

It is important to add that we do not always work this way. We would be putting too much of a constriction on ourselves. We often intervene right away, without the self-considering delay described above. If we paused before each of our interventions, the conversation with the client would lack immediacy. We can conceive of the moments when we react immediately as sliding down a much travelled path. This is also necessary, in order for us to get to know these habitual field movements firsthand. But then, at certain key moments, we implement the described speed bumps. How to recognize these key moments is further elaborated in Chapter 10, "Inviting a Stranger."

Countermovement of the Mind

How can we use the aforementioned general principles specifically when working with depression? Let us revisit the results of the study on the experiences of therapists during psychotherapy sessions with depressed clients (Roubal & Řiháček, 2016), this time from the perspectives of field theory and paradoxical change theory. It will require us to constantly defocus our minds. To resist the tendency to focus on individuals and their interactions. Instead, we will attempt to tune into field movements that transcend the beings participating in the given situation.

In live contact, the present moment is born from the previous one and gives birth to the next one. The situation naturally moves from *now for the next* (Spagnuolo Lobb, 2013). In depression, such a natural flow of the situation is blocked, smothered. The situation does not move. Nevertheless, the current is present with all its force, it just moves in a whirlpool of depression, thereby deepening the depression.

What blocks and knots the flow of the situation? The hungry desire for relational closeness can give us a hint. The desire for the closeness of another, during which one feels that they are alive. A depressive situation likely encompasses the fear that such an experience of closeness to another will never happen again. It is an existential, bodily-experienced abandonment. The horror of being completely alone in a world that is dead, unfeeling, empty. Something like a nightmare of a baby born into a cold void.

This abysmal emptiness is probably hidden in every situation, even in a naturally flowing one. It represents the flipside of the opportunity to meet another. Usually, however, it is mercifully covered by a naturally felt hope and only occasionally flashes through, for example, in the form of existential anxiety. However, in a depressive situation, the experience of hope is absent and thus does not protect against the experience of existential abysmal emptiness. This emptiness may then seem extremely threatening. It confronts people with the real possibility that the very basis of the lived human experience – that is, being able to relate to others – could disappear. That seems so profoundly existentially threatening and incites such terror that it is impossible to face head on.

We can imagine that the flow of the situation dodges the experience of such terror. The field organizes itself into a form that allows one to avoid directly experiencing abysmal emptiness. Yet this experience is only the flipside of the coin, the other being a live encounter. By turning away from the experience of an abandoned emptiness, one unfortunately also turns away from the possibility of meeting another person. Such avoidance of liveliness then further spins the whirlpool of depression. And the whirlpool pulls down more and more. That leads to another terrifying abandonment that the field organization was originally meant to avoid. A rescue attempt only intensifies the sinking. Such a hopeless cycle of the situation shapes the client and they express it outwardly with depressive symptoms.

Such cycling of the therapeutic situation also shapes us. As therapists, it probably comes naturally to us to help a person drowning in depression and at least give them some relief. In this way, through the natural effort to help, the whirlpool of depression can begin to suck us in. We thereby take on ourselves the responsibility for change, for a certain therapeutic outcome. We take on the responsibility of helping the suffering person in front of us. We can imagine this experience of responsibility as a kind of hook by which the whirlpool of depression of the situation grabs us and continues to drag us down.

As it is, depression does not usually alleviate during a session. We therapists can choose to take responsibility for that. Then we get frustrated with ourselves and we blame ourselves for our incompetence. Alternatively, we can attribute responsibility to the client and then get frustrated with them. We then accuse them (in our minds, not to them outright), of not trying hard enough: *"Actually (...) I'm angry. (...) With him. I could kick him!"* In both cases, frustration and aggression appear in the field. These are emotions that drive the therapist and the client apart. This can lead to exactly what the client feared most: they find themselves abandoned in a situation of unspoken frustration and aggression. So even here, in a therapeutic situation, the hopelessly abandoned emptiness deepens. And even here, there is an avoidance of directly experiencing it. Avoidance, which also entails a deflection from live contact between client and therapist. The whirlpool of depression continues to spin.

Hope Offered by the Situation

At precisely this moment, the field theory perspective offers us unexpected hope. We see depression as a movement of the situation, as a dynamic that organizes the field including the client and us. Such a view frees us from feeling responsible for change. Therefore, it frees us from responsibility for the result. At the same time, it allows us to stay with and in the ongoing process. To be open to what appears in a given situation – this is, in fact, the responsibility with which the field theory perspective entrusts us. We do not assume responsibility for the result, but we accept responsibility for how we are present in the process of change.

In depression, the natural flow of the situation is distorted, but it is still present as a possibility to which we as therapists can open the door. We can do so by taking on a strange, paradoxical approach: not feeling responsible for helping the suffering person in front of us, but at the same time, responding to their existential desire for the presence of another.

Such an approach can be the first step out of the whirlpool of depression. As therapists, we need to let go of our expectations while maintaining hope. Surrender to the "in-between" (Yontef, 1993) and follow the hidden wisdom of the situation itself. However, this is by no means a passive surrender. It is a very active process of freeing ourselves from the various expectations we have of ourselves and the client, and offering purified, simple and true presence.

However, offering a *meeting without aiming* (Yontef, 1993) is particularly difficult in a depressive situation, because therapists must resist the natural physically experienced survival instincts. Instincts that force both client and therapist to use any possible means to avoid the direct experience of the horror of the abandoned void. Yet paradoxically, following these survival instincts would only further strengthen the whirlpool of depression.

Thus, in order to escape from this whirlpool, we must likewise proceed paradoxically. In order to stay lively in contact with another in a depressive situation, we need to go against our survival instincts. We need to take an unnatural turn within ourselves into horror, into abandonment, into an abysmal void. As if when trapped in a life-threatening underwater current, we stopped fighting for air, stopped trying to surface. Instead, we give up, relinquish our fight, sink to the bottom, and there we paradoxically escape the downward-pulling power of the whirlpool.

Such surrendering is an active liberation from the physically experienced survival instincts. The client is too exhausted from long suffering to make such a countermovement. Therefore, as therapists, we must do it first. It is necessary for us to experience and survive the horror in the therapeutic situation. In order to revive hope in a situation, hope that such an unnatural movement against survival instincts is possible to survive.

Thus it is necessary for us to start with ourselves, to set our minds in the direction opposite to that which our survival instincts would have us take. This will change the way we are present with the client, how we sit with them and from where we make our intervention.

Establishing the countermovement of the mind is about immersing ourselves as therapists in the horror of a depressive situation as we encounter it in our own experience of powerlessness, hopelessness and exhaustion. In doing so, we create a basic premise for change. In our countermovement, we disrupt the cyclical pattern by which the depressive situation is organized.

As a result, we do not act out the usual response to depression (*depressed mood induction and rejection*) (Coyne, 1976) that only further reinforces depression in relationships outside of therapy. We do not follow the first impulse triggered by the fear of emptiness and the desire to change the depressive situation: *"It leads me to look for a solution."* Again, we would only further strengthen the depressive field organization by doing this.

Instead, we do what seems completely unnatural and even dangerous in the given situation. We remain open and receptive so that we can directly meet the fear deeply experienced in our own body and venture into it. By redirecting our reaction, we help redirect the flow of the situation. The current, which has been cyclically deepening the depression, begins to look for a new direction. Perhaps then it will gradually begin to erode the obstacles to the natural flow of the situation and move toward experiencing grieving.

As therapists, we can also invite grieving through ourselves. We can painfully and sorrowfully experience our powerlessness. Experience how limited we are in a given situation. Admit that everything is not in our power. We grieve all this and let it go with the pain. We surrender. The depressive situation dynamics, which we ourselves experience as exhaustion, frustration, powerlessness and hopelessness, guide us beautifully to come to terms with the reality of the current situation, with its stillness:

> *I realise (...) that it is my haste or precipitance or heaviness, that I want it quickly [to change]... So [I start doing it differently and] I'm still there [with him] (...) and I'm more silent.*

We stop trying to change something, we let go of our helper's role. This opens up the capacity for us to truly experience the presence of the other. The hope that the experience of being close to another is possible begins to revive:

> *It was a relief... It was quite a relief actually to feel that [improving depression] was not just some duty. (...) That actually for her the meeting [in itself] (...) has some kind of positive benefit. (...) So that actually helped me quite a bit."*

The meeting itself begins to make sense to us.

Thus, through us, the experience of hope and meaning comes to life in the depressive situation and can even flash through into the client's experience. In rare moments, like a suddenly and briefly sparkling star in the dark night sky, the client may also feel the true presence of the other. Feel the whiff of an encounter. Feel that we are here with them. As therapists, we experience relief at that moment, sometimes even with a touch of joy. This bodily-felt and freeing relief is a valuable signal for us that the natural *intentionality* of the situation is being unleashed and that there is a chance for restoring the natural flow. Hope emerges directly from the depressive situation.

Via this bodily experienced relief, our body then enjoys this freeing potential of the depressive situation. It receives support against being pulled into the whirlpool of depression:

Well, I feel that it helps me... when those moments of deeper contact occur. Because I start to perceive it as at least a little meaningful and somehow through it I can like that person even with all that. It helps, that there is not only that darkness, but also, something alive. Something really alive. [It helps me] that there is not only death there (...) [but also] there's life there... That when I got close to her, I felt not only her depression, but also her as a being.

But again, we have to be very careful not to scare hope away. Not to expect such moments to happen. We can only prepare the conditions for them, but we cannot make them come. That means that most of the time we sit in hopelessness. Outwardly, no change is visible. Only in ourselves, in our experience, relief appears because we have relinquished our efforts for a change. We have stopped trying to change the situation, we have accepted it as it is. And it is heavy, cold, empty:

It was like coming to stand firmly on the ground. Landing. You stop being involved in some activity there, but you just sit down. So you sit, [but] that wall is impenetrable. For one, it's a relief from the activity, but for the other, you're sitting there in something like, bad.

So far, the change has only taken place in our *mind-body set*. Although invisible, this change creates the basis for change that will be able to take place deep below the symptoms of depression. In the dynamics by which the field organizes. As therapists, we are now present differently because we are attuned to the intentionality of the situation, to the movement that is present as a healing possibility.

The way of our embodied residing in a situation has undergone a transformation. We do not try to change the situation, we do not cure depression, we do not push the river. Instead, we provide support to ourselves and thus set ourselves free. We stop limiting ourselves by reacting to the fear of being pulled into the whirlpool of depression. Our free position will then allow us to be receptive to the hidden potential of the depressive situation, to the movement that wants to happen. How we are present allows us to be transformed by this movement and thereby bring it to life.

Notes

1 For a given moment, we allow what we do together (ego function) and who we are for each other (personality function) to recede into the background.
2 The paradoxical theory of change is based both on the Western humanistic-existential psychotherapeutic tradition and on inspiration from Eastern philosophies, especially Zen Buddhism. It originally described the process of personal development, later it was developed as an overarching concept for the Gestalt therapeutic approach when working with clients (e.g. Philippson, 2005; Yontef, 2005).

Bibliography

Beisser, A. (1970). The paradoxical theory of change. In Fagan, J., Shepherd, L. (Eds.), *Gestalt therapy now*. Harper Colophon Books, 77–80.

Coyne, J. C. (1976). Toward an interactional description of depression. *Psychiatry*, 39, 28–40.

Francesetti, G., Roubal, J. (2020). Field theory in contemporary Gestalt therapy, Part 1: Modulating the therapist's presence in clinical practice. *Gestalt Review*, 24(2), 113–136.

Francesetti, G., Gecele, M., Roubal, J. (2013). Gestalt therapy approach to psychopathology. In Francesetti, G., Gecele, M., Roubal, J. (Eds.), *Gestalt therapy in clinical practice: From psychopathology to the aesthetics of contact*. FrancoAngeli, 59–76.

Grossman, D. (1989). *See under: LOVE*. Farrar, Straus and Giroux, p. 138.

Perls, F., Hefferline, R. F., Goodman, P. (1951). *Gestalt therapy: Excitement and growth in the human personality*. Julian Press.

Philippson, P. (2005). The paradoxical theory of change: Strategic, naive and Gestalt. In *Gestalt therapy: Roots and branches – Collected papers*. Karnac Books, 159–166.

Roubal, J., Francesetti, G. (2022). Field theory in contemporary Gestalt therapy. Part 2: Paradoxical theory of change reconsidered. *Gestalt Review*, 26(1), 1–33.

Roubal, J., Řiháček, T. (2016). Therapists' in-session experiences with depressive clients: A grounded theory. *Psychotherapy Research*, 26(2), 206–219.

Spagnuolo Lobb, M. (2013). *The now-for-next in psychotherapy: Gestalt therapy recounted in post-modern society*. FrancoAngeli.

Yontef, G. (1993). *Awareness, dialogue and process: Essays on Gestalt therapy*. Gestalt Journal Press.

Yontef, G. (2005). Gestalt therapy theory of change. In Woldt, A., Toman, S. (Eds.), *Gestalt therapy: History, theory, and practice*. Sage, 81–100.

Chapter 9

Above All, Get Out of the Way

We can imagine that we have now attuned our way of being in a depressive situation to support the flow of emerging dynamics. We have thus prepared the ground for us to actively intervene. Until now, we have been slowing ourselves down in a refined fashion and instead of intervening with the client, we have worked on ourselves. Although we might have been tempted to do something, we first attended to our own way of being in the therapeutic situation.

Returning briefly to the theory of the self as a process with three functions, we recall that the self can sound like a melody played by, say, these three instruments – flute, piano and bass. What we do (*ego function*), who we are (*personality function*) and how we are (*id function*). Until now, we have paid a lot of attention to how to be in a depressive situation (*id function*) and we have deliberately avoided what the urgency of the situation tempts us to, i.e. what we should do (*ego function*). So we can imagine that by first transforming our way of being, we strengthened the existential foundation of the depressive situation (the bass holds the rhythm). And now we can listen to what melody the flute will play (what we will do as therapists).

We have managed to maintain a creative tension between being and doing (Greenberg & Brownell, 1996), between the Eastern focus on conscious being and the Western emphasis on active doing (Melnick, Nevis & Shub, 2005). Perhaps now is the time to address the question that we have pushed aside until now: what can we do in a situation with a depressed client? What can we do now that we have established ourselves in a free and grounded position from which our interventions will emerge?

There are, of course, many different options for intervening in the complex experiential terrain of a depressive situation. An active intervention can be any of our decisions that we choose to implement in the given moment. A question, a smile, a comment, listening...

Essentially, it's perhaps possible to describe only the general purpose of psychotherapeutic work with depression. Where to aim. Thereafter, certain more loose guidelines can be offered to give direction to our interventions. These will guide each therapist in their specific selection and timing of their interventions. The situation will guide them. It is similar to stepping on uneven ground when walking. The foot adapts itself to the current ground, there is no need to think it through in detail in advance. But being present is necessary.

DOI: 10.4324/9781003500148-10

The basic *intention* is not to stand in the way of hope that is implicitly present in an encounter and to make room for change, which may come in its own way and its own time. This intention may seem strange from the point of view of contemporary Western medicine and psychotherapy focused on reducing symptoms. In principle, however, it is "a very traditional approach as per the old Taoist advice: don't stand in the way" (Perls, Hefferline & Goodman, 1951, p. 24). We can imagine that we do not make change. We just open the door for it. We open the door for it with every intervention, from which we expect nothing.[1]

What to Do in Depression

Above all, let us not stand in the way. And when we do something, let there not be too much of it. Laura Perls (2005, in Bloom, 2003) put it well: give as much support as needed and as little as necessary. So, keeping the *intention* described above, we can now get inspired by the framework guidelines for what to do in a depressive situation:

Just endure. We consciously choose to endure. And we support ourselves to make it through.[2] Depression affects the perception of both client and therapist. As therapists, we are a function of a field arranged in a depressive way and our experience is distorted by it, which then affects our judgment. As a result, it may seem to us that there is no chance of change, that the client's depression will last forever. But from a distance, the reality looks different. The deepest period of a depressive episode can last, for example, for two months. It is, of course, a very long and rough time for the client. But for us therapists, this might mean only eight sessions. That is something we can manage to endure. We can also remind ourselves that a therapy session, even though it might seem endless, has a limited timeframe. After all, we have the capacity to endure the 50 minutes and then step out of the depressively arranged field.

Enduring does not mean resigning and disconnecting. It does not even mean gritting your teeth and pushing yourself by sheer force of will to the end of the session. It just means persevering. Distributing energy as one would on a long hike. When we try too hard to pull the client out of the whirlpool of depression, we both just slide deeper down. On the other hand, we are not passive – that would also drag us down. We must fully concentrate on where we stand and what we are holding on to. We can anchor ourselves outside of the current therapeutic relationship by remembering what has helped in therapy with other depressed clients. We realize that we have faced a similar situation before and had the capacity to endure it. And we might also create a certain meaningful concept which will help us grasp the current situation. For example, we can realize that the client has recently started taking antidepressants. For us, this probably means that the therapist's task is now limited to supplementing the pharmacological treatment and supporting the client before the antidepressants start to work. Later on, therapy can have more ambitious goals, but at the moment, striving for higher goals would only increase feelings of frustration and powerlessness.

In this way, we pull ourselves out of shared timelessness and hopelessness. We are aware of the context of the current situation and anchor it in time and space: this is the therapy room, we meet here as therapist and client, our meeting lasts a certain limited time, the next meeting will be in a week. Such self-anchoring will allow us to endure and at the same time not be absorbed by the situation when time and space disappear in the whirlpool of depression (Francesetti & Roubal, 2013).

With this attitude, we also contribute to the transformation of the shared field. The field now ceases to organize solely in a depressive way of functioning, however much depression is in the foreground at the given moment. We therapists bring ourselves into the situation and transform it. By supporting ourselves in various ways, we emphasize the neglected aspect of self-support in a depressed situation. The possibility of supporting oneself then also actualizes for the client.

We simply try to do with the client what makes sense to us based on our knowledge, experience and intuition. At the same time, we know this is a marathon, not a sprint. We are aware that we can only invest a moderate amount of effort at a time, in order to be able to endure in the long run. The important thing is to endure. We can be inspired by the already mentioned saying: "Nature heals and the doctor amuses the patient in the meantime."

In regard to our relationship with the client, we balance in an unstable position, on the borderline between falling into shared depression and experiential detachment, between fusion (*confluence*) and isolation. Here, basic guardrails appear that define what would probably not be a good idea to do in a depressed situation. In principle, when carrying out specific interventions, it is necessary not to experientially detach from the client, but also not to fuse with them. In all likelihood, it will happen anyway. But when we notice that it has indeed happened, we need to realize that we slipped up, went too far and are already outside the domain of useful interventions.

How do we recognize this? In the case of detachment, we can most likely see that we are trying to pull the client out of depression with our interventions. We deliver optimism, we deliver liveliness, we stir, we push. We polarize ourselves against the client. In the case of fusion, on the other hand, we can probably recognize it in the fact that when our interventions fail, we lose self-awareness, we identify with our experiences. *"I feel incompetent, and that means I'm incompetent – as a therapist, as a person."* We pull the rug from under our own feet.

Within these guardrails, we therefore focus on our own firm stance and persistently offer a hand toward the client drowning in the swamp of depression. That is enough. The client can hold on to this stable and non-invasive contact and stop making desperate, futile and exhausting attempts to climb out of the swamp as quickly as possible. This will allow them to gradually gain strength and look for support points that they can lean on later in the next step of their journey up from depression. As Michael (from the previous chapter) said, when he emerged from several weeks of depression: *"I wasn't really noticing what you were doing with me. But it was nice that you were still here and still trying. Even when it didn't work."*

Explore. Simple exploration sounds easy, but it is not very easy in a depressed situation. Our natural reaction is likely to lead us to escape the depressive field by offering help. Instead, we look curiously and attentively into depression. What is important here is who we are with the client (*personality function*). We need to let the piano play louder. We are not rescuers, but explorers. We do not offer a rescue mission, but a map. We take interest in what the landscape of the client's life looks like. We notice with interest the little things that together compose the overall picture. Through simple, down-to-earth questions, firmer outlines emerge from the depressive boundless grey fog. *"What time did you wake up today? Have you been out today? And what did you do outside?'*

More bounded questions are better, ones that can be answered simply and concretely. This will allow the client to mobilize at least their remaining strength and invest it in contact with us. When the question is too open (*"How are you today?"*), contemplating and answering it requires too much strength which the client does not have. They cannot answer and they thus blame themselves for failing even in such a simple matter. In this way, we risk strengthening the whirlpool of depression even with just an overly demanding question.

Expand. The person before us is showing us how their world is hopelessly, painfully empty. Fundamentally important movements of the situation can then be started by a simple question from our side: *"How long has it been going on like this?"* We do not comfort or divert with such a question. We show interest, get closer, and also offer the client the opportunity to answer shortly and specifically, to not feel they have failed when answering. The concrete answer then begins to structure and fill the elusive void.

Thanks to this, time can start to flow, the perception of which is missing in depression. We can further support this: *"Have you ever experienced such a state before?" "And how long did it last then?"* By merely naming the fact that this consuming hopeless state lasted for a certain limited time can bring implicit hope to the current situation. It ended then. But again, we must not scare away hope with optimism. It is enough to leave it unsaid. If we push too hard for change (*"You see, it will also end now"*), the client will polarize against us and toward hopelessness.

Instead, we can make use of the polarization and deliberately go into the darkness. *"What was the worst thing about it then?" "Why do you think it lasted so long?"* We show that we are not afraid and are willing to stay with the client in their ordeal. Moreover, if we stay in this dark, inert polarity with the client, they themselves may after some time bring the other polarity, the desire for change. *"It was really horrible. I never want to experience that again. That's actually why I'm here…"*

We expand the perception of time, space, context. We ask what happened in the client's life when the depression started. And what was life like before? How did the depression develop, transform? Sometimes we can help transform how the client perceives their state. From being stuck in a black hole to sliding down a wave. We can physically demonstrate a downward movement with our hand: *"This is where you started to fall into depression and this is how you were sinking down into it. Yes?"* And then, for example, we can indicate with our hand the movement of the wave as it crests back up. *"Where are you now, approximately?"* When a client says, *"It's terrible right now, I'm at the bottom,"* we can indicate the place on the wave, *"so down here, all the way at the bottom?"* without trying to change it. Even this characterization brings implicit hope. If they are the lowest point now, things can only go slowly up again.

But we must not scare the hope away. We must not drag it into the light, but let it operate silently in the dark and maybe it will emerge on its own in time. What is important is our exploratory position: interest and acceptance of what is. The phenomenological naming of the current state itself *is intrinsically potent* (Melnick & Nevis, 2018). Just by situating the client's present experience within the dynamic concept of an experiential wave, we help start the flow of time again. We do not draw outside hope into the depressed situation, but only pay attention to what is present in the background of the situation. As such, hitherto neglected aspects of the situation can come to the foreground. We thus open the door to hope, which is already implicitly present.

Test the terrain. As we expand and explore, we may find that different parts of the client's landscape are variously firm. Most of the time, the answers we obtain from the client are not good launching pads, they do not help us further propel the conversation. It is like stepping on a certain point and discovering that there is depressive mud that gives way underfoot. Never mind, we did not expect much anyway, we did not lean into it that much. So we can try another point. We gradually discover that in the swamp of depression there are places that hold more firm, where we can hold a conversation with the client for a little while longer. For example, with one client, I talk about trees. This topic tangibly allows me to stand on firmer ground for a while.

We do not stay silent, without movement for long. Our own weight would drag us down into the depressive swamp. However, we do not expect that the conversation we are having with the client will lead to any improvement. If we tried to jump out of the depressive swamp like that, we would only sink deeper into it, our disappointment of failure would drag us further down. Instead, we grope horizontally in the conversation for solid footholds. Like feeling for stones to step on in the swamp of depression. It is not the content of what we talk about with the client that is important, but this, our aesthetic impression during the conversation. It leads us.

Welcome liveliness. We can also use our aesthetic perception of the situation to recognize how lively different aspects of the situation are. In a depressively organized field, perception changes in a specific way. Aspects of the situation that have a numbing or even deadening effect come to the foreground, while the enlivening aspects of the situation recede into the background. A common experience of depressed people is that they perceive the world as empty and grey. Only then, when they emerge from their depression, do they suddenly see colors around them again. Only then do the enlivening aspects of the situation come to the fore once again.

During a psychotherapy session, together with the clients, we experience a descent into emptiness, greyness and deadness. If we realize that this deadness is only one side of the situation, it helps us focus on aspects that have been in the background until now. But again, we do not try to change the situation by bringing liveliness from the outside (*"But look, it's already spring outside"*). Such encouragement would have the opposite effect on the client (*"Well, I can't enjoy it..."*). Instead, we focus on the liveliness that is already present in the therapeutic situation, albeit in the background. We find liveliness directly in the situation, in ourselves, in the client and in the therapeutic relationship. We can feel that some of the topics we discuss with the client bring at least a slight enlivenment. Or sometimes it warms up and enlivens the atmosphere when we make tea for ourselves and the client. Other times, enlivenment comes when we share our own ordinary everyday experience with the client. Again, it is not the content of what we talk about that is decisive, but the aesthetic quality of how we talk about it together.

Focus on the relationship. When we give up trying to change depression and focus on the therapeutic relationship, we redirect our attention away from the inanimate symptoms and toward the client as a living being. Bringing the relationship to the foreground is a key moment in creating a solid base for therapist and client to lean on in the midst of the whirlpool of depression.

How to focus on the therapeutic relationship? Simply by awakening, in ourselves, an interest in the client as a person. We decide to participate in a *meeting without aiming* (Yontef, 1993). This alone brings the relationship to the fore without us necessarily having to talk about it.

Every now and then, we can also show ourselves more as a living person. *"It seems to me that when I'm experiencing powerlessness and tiredness here now, I can actually taste what you live with all the time. It helps me to imagine how difficult it must be for you."* We can use our own experience in this way to reach out to the client across the abyss of depressive emptiness. The client can then hopefully feel that we see and understand them. Perhaps only for a brief moment. But even that revives hope in the situation. Hope that reaching the other does not have to be completely impossible and hopeless. But we still have to be careful from where this intervention arises. If we need to say it for our own sake, it is better to remain silent.

It may seem that the therapeutic process is stagnant and the symptoms remain the same. But this can also be understood as the therapeutic process simply not going the way of improving depressive symptoms. Instead, it takes a different path for the moment: the therapeutic relationship deepens, thereby building the necessary relational foundation for change. Therefore, if the client's depression does not change in therapy, we can welcome this as a warning that the relational base needs to be strengthened. The need for a relationship becomes a figure, which must be prioritized over trying to change the symptoms of depression.

Slow down and attract change. Lastly, here a possible intervention that we once again aim back at ourselves as therapists. When we feel the tendency to act quickly, let us slow down. In this way, we not only invite change, we even try to attract it. But this is a big topic deserving of the entire following chapter.

Notes

1   The intention of interventions is therefore not to bring about change, but to accept reality and support the movement that is about to happen. The decision of how to go about this is based on an aesthetic criterion based directly on the current situation (intrinsic) (Bloom, 2003; Francesetti, 2012; Roubal, Gecele & Francesetti, 2013). We then choose our intervention based on a holistic perception of the forces present at a given moment (phronesis) (Francesetti, 2019; Francesetti & Roubal, 2020).
2   A qualitative study on this topic (Ebertová, 2016) described the following coping strategies of therapists when working with depressed clients: conceptualizing of the situation in a larger context, focusing on one's own needs, physical anchoring, slowing down, recognizing the limits of one's own responsibility.

Bibliography

Bloom, D. J. (2003). Tiger! tiger! burning bright: Aesthetic values as clinical values in Gestalt therapy. In Spagnuolo, M. L., Amendt-Lyon, N. (Eds.), *Creative license: The art of Gestalt therapy*. Springer Verlag, 63–78.

Ebertová, L. (2016). *Zvládající strategie terapeutů při práci s depresivními klienty.* Diplomová práce. [*Coping strategies of therapists when working with depressed clients.* Thesis.] Masaryk University, Brno.

Francesetti, G. (2012). Pain and beauty: From psychopathology to the aesthetics of contact. *British Gestalt Journal*, 21(2), 4–18.

Francesetti, G. (2019). The field strategy in clinical practice: Towards a theory of therapeutic phronesis. In Brownell, P. (Ed.), *Handbook for theory, research and practice in Gestalt therapy* (2nd ed.). Cambridge Scholars Publishing, 268–302.

Francesetti, G., Roubal, J. (2020). Field theory in contemporary Gestalt therapy, Part 1: Modulating the therapist's presence in clinical practice. *Gestalt Review*, 24(2), 113–136.

Greenberg, L. S., Brownell, P. (1996). Validating Gestalt. *Gestalt!*, 1(1). www.academia. edu/28055225/Validating_Gestalt_An_Interview_with_Leslie_Greenberg

Melnick, J., Nevis, S.M. (2018). *The evolution of the Cape Cod model. Gestalt conversations, theory, and practice.* Gestalt Therapy Book Series. Istituto di Gestalt HCC Italy Publ.

Melnick, J., Nevis, S. M., Shub, N. (2005). Gestalt therapy methodology. In Woldt, A. L., Toman S. M. (Eds.), *Gestalt therapy: History, theory, and practice.* Sage Publications, 101–115.

Murakami, H. (2017). *Men without women.* Knopf, p. 55.

Perls, F., Hefferline, R. F., Goodman, P. (1951). *Gestalt therapy: Excitement and growth in the human personality.* Julian Press.

Roubal, J., Gecele, M., Francesetti, G. (2013). Gestalt therapy approach to diagnosis. In Francesetti, G., Gecele, M., Roubal, J. (Eds.), *Gestalt therapy in clinical practice: From psychopathology to the aesthetics of contact.* FrancoAngeli, 79–106.

Yontef, G. (1993). *Awareness, dialogue and process: Essays on Gestalt therapy.* Gestalt Journal Press.

Chapter 10

Inviting a Stranger

What is psychopathology? The existential pain and suffering we experience in life due to various limitations and losses is not psychopathology (Salonia, 2013; Francesetti, 2019a). Psychopathology begins when a person cannot process and integrate the experiences they have in a difficult situation because they lack the other whose presence would make this possible (Francesetti, 2019a, 2021; Francesetti & Roubal, 2020).

The other whom one would need to process a difficult, painful experience is missing. The person thus remains alone with their experience. Without the support of another, they cannot grasp it, experience it or even feel it. Their experience remains chaotic and disorganized on an undifferentiated physical level. But a person can defend themselves against such chaos in various ways. For example, one strategy is putting unprocessed experiences aside, where they are as little bother as possible. Dissociated in this way, the experiences then park themselves in place, shaped into packages of symptoms and syndromes. Psychiatric diagnostic systems describe various forms of such packages.

Psychopathologies of assorted forms are therefore, from this point of view, the result of the human ability to creatively adapt to what could not be fully experienced and processed. It could be said that psychopathology is the trace of one who is missing (Francesetti, 2019a, 2021; Francesetti & Roubal, 2020). And also the way they are missing. And what we needed them to be for us.

So we see psychopathology as a form of creative adaptation to the absence of the other. The experience of missing the other at the moment when they were needed is transformed and thus present in the psychopathology that we as therapists encounter with the client. And it is in this way that the missing other becomes present even in the therapeutic relationship in the here and now. The client is sort of paralyzed, blinded, deadened. This is how they have survived alone, without the support of the other. This is also the way they relate to us in the therapy session. Through psychopathology, we therapists thus meet the one who is missing.

In an aesthetic perception of contact with the client, we can get a sense for what is missing, like traces in the dark, like drops of emptiness. During the flow of the therapeutic process, there are certain moments when it seems as though something gets stuck or skips a beat, as if something is lacking for the fluency. These

DOI: 10.4324/9781003500148-11

moments of absence (Francesetti, 2019a, 2021; Francesetti & Roubal, 2020) point to experiences that the client could not experience, process and integrate into their life story. Therefore, the client cannot differentiate themselves from these experiences (which have not yet happened) and they are thus only covertly present in the client's way of being in the world. Due to this, they are also present with us in the therapeutic process.[1] Both client and therapist experience these absences as forces that try to happen, become present, *become embodied*. We experience these forces, for example, as fleeting impressions, elusive physical sensations or a holistically perceived atmosphere (Francesetti & Griffero, 2019).

In this way, we experience on ourselves the *intentionalities of the field*, which strive for the kind of contact that would loosen stuck dynamics. The psychopathologically formed situation could then begin to transform into a continuous, subsequent stream of present moments. It could move toward a freer flow of the situation, in which participants really see one another, can express themselves to one another and can also be open to the other's reactions. And toward a situation where its participants would be continuously transformed by experiencing the flow of live contact.

Letting Yourself Be Disturbed

Let us return one last time to the study on the experience of psychotherapists in a depressive situation (Roubal & Řiháček, 2016), this time perhaps to the most intriguing aspect of the results: how is it possible that the therapist can completely lose themselves.

> As I get closer to him in those emotions, closer to the client, [there is] a limit where I [say in my mind to the client:] 'You should go see a psychologist, man.' Before I realize that he is actually there [at the psychologist]! (...) I forget that I am there as a psychologist. Because I realize how hard it is for me when he describes it to me. And I think that's because of the closeness.[2]

This is the testimony of a therapist in a psychotherapy situation. Depression can suck us in so much that we lose track of who we are in the situation. In a depressively organized field, we begin to lack our own liveliness, creativity and competence. Who we are there changes. We lose ourselves.

The dynamics of the depressive situation thus transform not only the client, but also us therapists. We are both a function of the depressed field in the here and now. Again, we can imagine the depressive field as a mycelium, omnipresent and at the same time hidden beneath the surface, invisible and undetectable. From this field, mushrooms grow visible above the surface: the client's symptoms of clinical depression and the therapist's experiences of hopelessness, powerlessness and incompetence. The fact that we lose ourselves in the depressive field is also a manifestation of this field. What if we did not fight it and used it instead? The situation itself shaped us this way. And we can lean on our understanding that the self is a function of the field movements. As a result, we need not try to get our competences back and get back into the saddle. Instead, we can try to submit to the process of losing ourselves,[3] not clinging to ourselves, letting ourselves be shaped in the flow of the transforming situation.

But it may be far from easy. We may not like what happens with us. Sometimes, we may not even want to see what is happening with us. And here comes the fundamentally important moment that invites us to participate in change. What do we not want to know about ourselves? What aspect of our current experience are we turning our eyes away from? At this moment, we have a chance to step out of the established pattern. Instead of looking away, we can try to look directly at our experience. Honestly yet inquisitively, with self-kindness. *"Powerlessness, anger. Feeling like it's pointless. It occurs to me that it would probably be good if he committed the suicide that he keeps talking about... That comes into my mind."* This is how one colleague describes how he completely lost empathy with his depressed client. At such a moment, he wants to get rid of the other person, he even seems to wish him dead.

Something like this can happen to us too. In a depressive situation, we might be frustrated and angry, we might lose empathy, we might want to be rid of the client. This is what really happens inside us, this is our inner reality. At such moments, it is important to accept the situation in its entirety, with all the associated experiences, including our own experience, from which we turn away. We can imagine such an experience as an unwelcome "stranger at the door" (Francesetti, 2019a, 2019b; Francesetti & Roubal, 2020).

As if our usual experiences were sitting quietly at home around the dinner table, surrounded by the light and warmth of a familiar home. Outside it is cold and windy and dark. We hear something like a knock on the door, probably someone wants us to let them in. Oh no! Don't disturb us now! We look away, we cover our ears, we do not want to let the contentment of how we are used to experiencing ourselves be disturbed. As if an experience of something we do not want to feel is being born inside us. Something we may see as senseless, strange. Something we might be ashamed of. It throws us off balance, it does not leave us in peace. Something out of place.[4] As if a stranger is trying to intrude on our usual experience. We feel a perfectly natural tendency to ignore them, not let them disturb us.

Instead, we can actually focus our attention on exactly what it is that we do not want to see with this particular client. We can invite the stranger in. We can open the door to what has no form, what has not yet had a chance to happen, what has no place here. And what at the same time tries to make itself present here and now in the therapeutic situation through our out-of-place experience.

The stranger appears at the nodal moments of the therapeutic process, which in these moments balances between transformation and repetition, between retraumatization and therapeutic change (Francesetti & Roubal, 2020). We cannot arrange these precious moments, but we can pave the way for them. We prepare the conditions for them during the entire therapeutic process, especially by building a safe and accepting environment, a trustworthy working alliance. It is as if the whole therapeutic process is a plant that we water and supply with nutrients, and that can blossom and bear fruit at these key moments.

So what is actually happening at such a moment? During a therapy session, experiences that could not be experienced intrude on the level of undifferentiated experience, at the level where the self and the environment are not yet separated. The experience thus cannot yet be attributed to me or to the other.[5] Such undifferentiated experiences seek ways to actualize, to happen. They want someone to bodily experience them so they can be integrated into story and memory. But the client's physical being is not enough for that, just as it was not enough for it in the past. The physical co-being of another is needed.[6] Ours.

We resonate with the *intentionality of the situation*. This resonance may come to us in the form of a feeling, a physical sensation or a pain, an image, a metaphor, a sound or a melody. Something that in a certain way deviates from our attunement to the client (Francesetti, 2015, 2019a). What we perceive on the periphery of our attention as something inappropriate or unacceptable.

The stranger who comes to us in this form tries to break out of the fixed, repetitive way of the field organization and provoke us therapists to an unexpected diversion from this pattern (Francesetti & Roubal, 2020). The weirder they seem to us, the more care we probably need to give them. Their strangeness suggests a degree of dissociation and thus determines how much our presence is needed. Their strangeness shows all that is at stake in that moment. The possibility of transforming the old pattern offers itself up. This can happen when we, through ourselves, allow the empty space to fill with an anticipating, unformed, unprocessed experience. On the other hand, there is also a great possibility of retraumatization. That can happen when, at this pregnant moment, we give in to the well-established, habitual movement and the situation turns back to the same old side again.

Second Wave

How do we know that this important moment in the therapy process has arrived? We will likely not know for sure. We will probably need to be able to tolerate a great deal of uncertainty. Follow hints without knowing where they lead. Rely on our cultivated sensitivity to the aesthetic quality of the ongoing process. We can liken it to being carried by a river and feeling the power of the current below the surface. As if we are sensing a general change in the atmosphere: we feel that something important may happen right now.

At such a moment, it is important to create a little more space for ourselves between the appearance of our experience-stranger and our intervention toward the client. (This door for transformation only opens for a moment. Nevertheless, if we outrun it, it will probably reappear. The stranger will try to get in again.) In the space we create, we work with ourselves.[7] Without expectations and without judging,[8] we pay attention to what is happening with us in a given situation. We slow down and wait to see what happens with us. How the field dynamics shape us. Whatever appears in our experiences, we must first simply notice it.

Realizing what we experience in the presence of a client is only the first, perhaps simpler step. The next step is what we do with this realization. How we face it. We can try not to criticize ourselves for our experience and instead observe it with curiosity (Evans & Gilbert, 2005). We can try to maintain a certain freely inquisitive attitude toward ourselves: *That's interesting, what strange things are happening to me now.* As if allowing ourselves to experience what is coming and at the same time not identifying with it: *I do not take what I feel personally.* As if letting our experience pass through us and perceiving it as a report about the field forces that shape us in a habitual, stereotypical way.

This then is how we encounter the *first wave* of our experience. If we intervene now, we are likely to avoid the anxiety stemming from what is emerging. If our activity toward the client is based on this first wave of our experience, we are likely to support the fixed pattern by which the psychopathological field repeatedly organizes. To illustrate, let us go back to Victor (see Chapter 7, "The Art of 'Doing Nothing'"). Here, we are halfway through the fourth session:

> Victor: "And she [the wife] just says: that's your fight now, I've got enough to deal with. She doesn't give a damn about me, so…"
>
> Therapist: "And what would you need from her?"
>
> "Oh nothing. I don't want anything from her. She lives her life, doesn't give a damn about me. I don't even blame her."
>
> "You know, it seems to me that it might be difficult for your wife to help you, maybe she doesn't know how. Perhaps you could give her a hint of what you need from her."
>
> "Sure, she's got it tough, having to live with me. Everyone stands up for her."
>
> (I want to continue the conversation, but I stop for a moment and notice what is happening. As if my eyes wanted to roll toward the ceiling in a gesture of angry resignation. My eyes want to, but I stop them. You can't do that! Aha, the stranger is here, I guess, so let's see what he says. What do I feel when I want to roll my eyes like that? Something like: "It's futile. Whatever I do is wrong. No matter how I try to get closer to Victor, he pushes me away.")
>
> If I were to express the first wave of my experience toward him, it would be something like this: "I've had enough. If you want to play the victim, then do it without me. I don't need this. I'm done with you." This first wave of my experience informs me of how the field usually organizes itself. It informs me of the power that is reshaping us both. My experience leads to rejection, devaluation and abandonment of the other. It is quite possible that others in Victor's presence also experience something similar, probably even his wife. And since others probably react to this first wave, Victor remains alone. That's why he came to therapy. He actually, through the first wave of my experience, clearly shows me what his problem is, why he came to me. It's not about me, I don't have to take it personally, I'm just familiarizing myself with a specific psychopathological pattern.

Here it is important that we stop and dissolve our quick instinctive reactions. That we wait a little longer for what appears next in our experience. That we wait for the second wave of our experience. By not reacting to the first wave, we have cleared the way for the second.[9]

So we let the first wave pass and wait to see what the second wave will bring to the shore. The second wave can appear thanks to our acceptance of the situation and thanks to the free curiosity with which we accept our own experiences of the first wave. We accept them and do not identify with them. This acceptance then enables change, as shown by the concept of the paradoxical theory of change (Beisser, 1970).

The second wave of our experience is usually accompanied by relief. We breathe easier when we are not crammed into the restrictively rigid pattern of the field organization. A sense of purpose emerges, although it may not yet take the form of any concrete thought. The situation has been unblocked and can move, although it may not yet be clear where. In addition to relief, the feelings that appear in the second wave can also be accompanied by joy, hope, lightness or even happiness. The feelings of the second wave themselves can be variable; they are often pity, tenderness or the feeling of being moved by something. We may not be entirely clear on what happened, but we sense possibilities opening up.

While the first wave of our experience informs us of the psychopathological field organization, the second wave brings an experiential report of what is missing. We can also read it as information about a relational need that was not fulfilled in the client's story (Evans & Gilbert, 2005). Only when we see the second wave in the context of the first can understanding begin to come and prepare us for active intervention. It is often an intuitive understanding, because there is not enough time in the session for logical construction. Together with a certain metaphor, image, sound or memory, what is happening suddenly begins to make sense. Let us return to the therapist and Victor:

It's best that I don't react to the first wave and wait to see what comes next.

What's coming? Mmmm, that's strange. My bottom lip curled up a little as if I wanted to cry. Not as an adult, but as a small child. And with that comes an image: I see Victor as a little boy in a sandbox. He wants to play with the others, but because he knocks down their sandcastles in the process, they all run from him. As an adult, I feel like sitting down in the sand with the abandoned and confused Victor: "Victor, look, this is how you made a sandcastle. See? Now you try. Try again. Yes, that's better. See? You did it. And now we'll try it together." I want to teach him to play with others. Okay, interesting second wave. So this is what he needed and didn't get? The first wave now makes sense in the context of the second. He needs someone who won't get mad at him for ruining their sandcastle. Someone who doesn't care about their own castles, but about Victor. Who wants to teach him how it's done when people are together.

But again, we can legitimately ask: *That's all well and nice, but what should I do at that moment?* Let us go back to the three functions of self. By inviting a stranger into our own experience, we have enriched the way we are present in a situation. We are more colorful, more variable, with more choices, more meaningful. In this way, we are present (*id function*) and based on it, we also start to relate to the client differently (*personality function*). We see not only what relational patterns he is stuck in and how he repeats them with us, but we also see a person longing for another, for the fulfillment of relational needs. That is why we are there with him. We become the one who can offer a new relational experience.

What to do then (*ego function*)? After all, we know that the situation will show us what to do, differently each time. It is important to endure the uncertainty, to relax in it. Let go of expectations, lean on ourselves. The main work is already done. The background of the situation is transformed and a new figure can grow out of it without us having to make any effort. However, I would like to mention two things we can do: self-disclosure and preparation.

Self-disclosure, i.e. a specific intervention where the therapist talks about themselves, is a very powerful tool. It needs to be handled with care and used judiciously.[10] The concept of two waves of experiences can be very helpful here. As long as we as therapists feel only the first wave, it is probably not a good idea to share it with the client. The first wave of our experience is part of a psychopathological dynamic, and by sharing it, there is a risk of retraumatization. But if we wait for the second wave of our experience, the two waves together will create a new dynamic. Together, they begin to make new meaning, and sharing our experience with the client can then open the way to working together on transforming the psychopathological field. Together, we can search for the meaning to which the dynamics between the first and second waves of experience point (Francesetti & Roubal, 2020). If we ourselves fail to meaningfully connect the first and second waves of our experience, it is better to wait, not to share our experience with the client. A meaningful connection may show itself to us later, in the next session or perhaps with the help of a supervision session.

Preparation. So we work with our experience by waiting for what comes after it. It is also important to pay enough attention to what precedes it. How we ourselves are ready for it. In order to be able to notice a stranger in our experiencing and to be able to capture the first and second waves of experience, it is necessary to make room for them in advance. We need to clean up our inner workplace before getting to work. We can do that on a macro level – taking some time for ourselves in the morning before a day with clients or practicing self-care a few minutes before a session with a particular client.

We can also do it on a micro-level: before saying something or even before feeling something. We can, in a moment, bodily prepare ourselves for what is to come, what we will experience in the next moment. If we begin to pick up signs that something is about to happen, we can work with attention. First, we focus it largely on ourselves, we prepare space in ourselves. It is about being able to really feel the experiences and simultaneously being so anchored in ourselves that we do not identify with them, we let them come and go. As if we let our experiences pass through us. We take care of the *fore-contact* part of the process (Perls, Hefferline & Goodman, 1951) in order to prepare a background which, when contact takes place, we can lean on and let ourselves be carried by the current.

The Stranger and the Waves in Depression

The two metaphors described – the stranger and the dual waves – can serve in general as guidelines for a therapist's work with their own experience. Their use is not tied specifically to work with depression. They can be used for generally psychotherapeutic work from the field theory perspective, regardless of the nature of the client's problems. The following case study fragment shows how these metaphors can be helpful in working with depression.

Susan is 74 years old and now experiences a "hopeless emptiness" in her life. She wakes up at half past three in the morning and then lies in bed until eleven, unable to get herself to move even to brush her teeth. She physically feels so weak that she is not even able to walk to the bathroom. She lies facing the wall, her head buried under the covers, a creeping, sticky pain running through her. As she says, "the loneliness is so palpable that it hurts."

What do I experience with her when she comes to psychotherapy sessions? A general heaviness. And something like, "Okay, someone like this again... Do I really want to listen to this?" And with that, "Hey, wake up! You are here to help her, so don't feel sorry for yourself and do something!" Aggressive disconnection associated with forced mobilization. Okay, I'll notice what I'm experiencing. It's the first wave, I'll wait for the second one. And I really have no idea what that could be.

What comes up is this: "Mmm, it's actually kind of weird. This lady seems too old to me to go to psychotherapy for the first time in her life. What brought her here anyway? I think it will be quite strange and quite special to work with such an old lady. What might her dreams and hopes for the future be? And what do I know, when she is almost thirty years older than me?!" Curiosity, challenge, humility. As if I somehow feel that she is special in some way. It's like I'm starting to be lured by exploring what's really going on with her and where it might go.

"Yes, yes. I hear how hard it must be for you right now." Should I follow the second wave of my experience and begin to take interest in what she is experiencing, what makes her experience special? "And could you tell me, what is it that hurts so much?" As I say this, I feel myself wade further into the depressive swamp. I'm going against the instinctive first reaction. I do not disconnect from the client, nor do I try to comfort her (to protect myself from co-experiencing depression). If I did, I would be letting her know that I don't want to let her suffering fully get to me.

When I ask "What is it that hurts so much?" Susan looks at me as if to make sure I'm serious. "I hate myself. I hate that I'm so useless... I say to myself: You're a lazy pig! ... Pull yourself together! You have to do something with yourself, it can't go on like this!" Hard look, hard face. I can feel the atmosphere stiffening. Her face represents an obstacle, it is like a stone that prevents the natural flow of the situation.

"Mmm, yes, I understand... And how does it feel now, when you say it to me like that?" I subtly point out that she is saying this to me, here and now. That

she's actually inviting me into her experience and I'm not running away, instead I'm slowly starting to get closer to her. "Well, I just feel that I'm useless. It's impossible! I have always, all my life, worked like a mule. No vacation, always work. That's how I was, I managed everything... And now I'm completely useless!"

Again, the boulder blocks the flow of the situation. I can feel the thick and still atmosphere full of hopelessness. But not completely. The moment I hear the words "no vacation," it's as if I hear a shiver of something else, as if something is awakening in my experience, some kind of timid (and inappropriate) sarcasm: "Really, no vacation in all those years?!" I perceive it as a hint of a well-hidden possibility. Is this the direction it would like to go in? A subtle hint of a direction? That hidden, precious moment was revealed to me through a subtle change in my experience. In the generally deadened atmosphere, I felt a revival at the words "no vacation" and let myself be guided by this hint.

I ask Susan about work. What did she do that she was working so hard?

"Oh, I always had at least two jobs. And always lots of energy. Now I'm so worn out..."

And there it is again: heaviness, hopelessness. Now it is important not to console and not to pull away. Take her suffering seriously: "Mmm... and would you tell me how you feel the tiredness?"

"I'm tired all the time. My body has no strength, I can't move. It takes me hours to get myself out of bed. I'm just useless."

Again I feel myself being pulled into the whirlpool of depression. No movement, her face like stone in the deadened atmosphere. And yet, when the word "body" was spoken, I felt another jolt of revival. What am I pushing away that I don't want to see? That's really weird. I wonder: what does her body look like? What does the body of a battered old lady look like? I find it very rude to look at her like that. A stranger, good and proper. Okay, so I'm not going to turn away from what I'm experiencing. I will not be deterred by feelings of shame and inappropriateness. I'll stick with it. Maybe the shame and inappropriateness is the first wave. I'll wait.

I still see the old body in front of me. Like from some old painting in chiaroscuro that emphasizes wrinkles and wear. A picture from some old master? An old master who could look at an old body and paint its beauty. Reverence and respect for the old body. The second wave.

Vacation and body. In my mind, these two hints of the aesthetic perception of the situation connect. Tremors of hope, that's how I perceive them. It's like jumping from one firmer place to another in a swamp. Vacation and body.

"Maybe your body is taking a vacation right now...?" She looks up, surprised. For a brief moment she seems to notice the living creature in front of her, to glimpse me.

We spend the rest of the session talking about what she did in her life and how she longed to be able to rest sometime. For it to be possible to relax. At the next session, she reports to me again that she spent the whole morning in bed, unable to get up. "But it's actually a bit different now," she says.

At that moment, I feel a flicker of hope with her, it feels a little stronger, I can feel it clearly now. As if a fresh breeze blew through the room. "How is it different?"

"Well, I don't move all morning, I stare at the wall, the covers over my head. I try to say to myself: There. Now I'm taking a vacation for all those years."

"And what is it like?"

"Still the same... I guess I'll try again, it's kind of weird..."

Nothing really changed. Susan is still depressed. Exhausted, unable to even get out of bed. But something is changing a little. Her approach to herself. That's actually quite a change from, "You're lazy as a pig!" to "I'm taking a vacation for all those years." She tried to stop blaming herself, insulting herself. She tried to redirect the fixed dynamics of the vicious cycle of depression that were draining her more and more. And instead she tried something new. Accepting the state she is in now. Legitimizing it. She began to learn how to be kind, compassionate to herself. The potential for it is there, she is lured to it and she's naturally led in that direction, she just needed another to bring that potential to life. Another human being who sees how battered she is and how she needs rest. Who will appreciate her work and the wisdom of her body.

It is clear that the fixed vicious cycle of depression is still far stronger. But we can see that Susan is attracted to the new "strange" idea that the body is now taking a vacation. It is possible to feel the hope of aliveness in it. In order to invite change, it is necessary to open up, and with our living presence support Susan in what is. Instead of running away from my own hopelessness, trying to help her and promoting my idea of what should be. By doing so, I would be standing in the way of a budding hope. Not standing in the way of hope – that is my task here and now. Hearing the small voice of hope in the roar of the sweeping whirlpool of depression. Seeing hope directly inside depression and not scaring it away with our own optimism.

We did one more thing to invite change in. We prepared a place for it to settle. A place defined by a new conceptualization of depression, a new grasp of the depressive experience. Instead of "I'm useless," it's "I'm taking a vacation." This new conception clears the way for the flow of the situation, a flow that is no longer blocked by harsh self-criticism, by the ossified stone. Instead of a depressing black hole, instead of the trap of the depressing whirlpool, a new image now emerges: a vacation after a lifetime of hard work. An idea that has its own dynamics. It is a place to which change is invited. Perhaps there, Susan will be able to experience the pain and regret over missed joys. To cry over them and let them go.

Notes

1 Francesetti calls these forces "proto-feelings" (Francesetti, 2019b, 2021; Francesetti & Roubal, 2020) and refers to Damasio (2012), who calls the first moments of the emerging self "proto-self." This is the first stage of something becoming reality, but it is not

yet formed and it is not yet possible to assign it to me or to the other, because this division appears later (Damasio, 2012).

2 The statements of therapists-participants in the mentioned study are again used in the text.

3 Fritz Perls (1992) argued that it is necessary to disintegrate in order to reintegrate. He was originally talking about the client, but we can also apply it to us therapists.

4 Francesetti also calls such disturbing experiences *atopon* (Francesetti, 2019a, 2019b) (from the Greek: that which is out of place).

5 Just because the therapist perceives that there are forces that affect them does not mean that it is the client affecting the therapist. From the field theory perspective, these forces belong to the situation as a whole. They arise from a whole that is qualitatively different from the sum of its parts, just as when a molecule of oxygen meets two molecules of hydrogen, a new quality of water is created (Francesetti & Roubal, 2020). From this point of view then, it makes no sense to try to distinguish between "what is mine" and "what is yours."

6 Here Francesetti (2019a, 2019b) refers to the philosophy of J. L. Marion. *Lending the flesh* (Marion, 2003) of the therapist is needed to set these processes of change in motion.

7 A detailed elaboration of the sequence of individual steps of working with oneself at this moment is offered by "Guidelines for Modulating the Therapist's Presence" (Francesetti & Roubal, 2020).

8 An approach inspired by Husserl's concept of "epoché" (Bloom, 2009, 2019).

9 To facilitate access for the second wave of our experience, we can ask ourselves: "What is it like for me to be experiencing what I am experiencing?" (Francesetti & Roubal, 2020).

10 Self-disclosure can be of two kinds – the therapist can share their own experience with the client or they can share something from their personal story. Here, we are concerned with sharing the therapist's own experience.

Bibliography

Beisser, A. (1970). The paradoxical theory of change." In Fagan, J., Shepherd, L. (Ed.), *Gestalt therapy now*. Harper Colophon Books, 77–80.

Bloom, D. J. (2009). The phenomenological method of Gestalt therapy: Revisiting Husserl to discover the essence of Gestalt therapy. *Gestalt Review*, 13(3), 277–295.

Bloom, D. J. (2019). Gestalt therapy and phenomenology: The intersection of parallel lines. In Brownell, P. (Ed.), *Handbook for theory, research, and practice in Gestalt therapy* (2nd ed.). Cambridge Scholars Publishing, 183–202.

Christensen, L. S. (2013). *The half brother*. Arcade, p. 506.

Damasio, A. (2012). *Self comes to mind: Constructing the conscious brain*. Vintage.

Evans, K., Gilbert, M. (2005). *An introduction to integrative psychotherapy*. Palgrave Macmillan.

Francesetti, G. (2015). From individual symptoms to psychopathological fields: Towards a field perspective on clinical human suffering. *British Gestalt Journal*, 24(1), 5–19.

Francesetti, G. (2019a). The field strategy in clinical practice: Towards a theory of therapeutic phronesis. In Brownell, P. (Ed.), *Handbook for theory, research and practice in Gestalt therapy* (2nd ed.). Cambridge Scholars Publishing, 268–302.

Francesetti, G. (2019b). A clinical exploration of atmospheres: Towards a field-based clinical practice. In Francesetti, G. A., Griffero T. (Ed.), *Psychopathology and atmospheres: Neither inside nor outside*. Cambridge Scholars Publishing, 35–68.

Francesetti, G. (2021). *Fundamentals of phenomenological-Gestalt psychopathology: A light introduction*. L'Exprimerie.

Francesetti, G., Griffero, T. (2019). Introduction. In Francesetti, G., Griffero, T. (Ed.), *Neither Inside Nor Outside. Psychopathology and atmospheres: Neither inside nor outside*. Cambridge Scholars Publishing, 1–5.

Francesetti, G., Roubal, J. (2020). Field theory in contemporary Gestalt therapy, Part 1: Modulating the therapist's presence in clinical practice. *Gestalt Review*, 24(2), 113–136.

Marion, J. L. (2003). *The erotic phenomenon*. University of Chicago Press.

Perls, F. (1992). *Gestalt therapy verbatim* (2nd ed.). Gestalt Journal Press.

Perls, F., Hefferline, R. F., Goodman, P. (1951). *Gestalt therapy: Excitement and growth in the human personality*. Julian Press.

Roubal, J., Řiháček, T. (2016). Therapists' in-session experiences with depressive clients: A grounded theory. *Psychotherapy Research*, 26(2), 206–219.

Salonia, G. (2013). Social context and psychotherapy. In Francesetti, G., Gecele, M., Roubal, J. (Ed.), *Gestalt therapy in clinical practice: From psychopathology to the aesthetics of contact*. FrancoAngeli, 189–199.

Chapter 11

Something for the Road

I mentioned at the very beginning, I write as if I am whittling a wood figure. The shape emerges gradually by carving away at the linden block from different sides. It seems to me that here, at the end of the book, the shape is quite visible. I would now like to try to highlight this shape and summarize what I consider substantial for a therapist's work with themselves in the presence of a depressed client.

We sit in front of the client on the therapist's chair. And since we are sitting, we take care of how we sit through it. How we manage ourselves to be able to sit through it. How to be well grounded and free in a depressing situation that pulls us in. It pulls us in, it is unpleasant and dangerous for us. It forces us to protect ourselves by trying to help the other. It tells us that with this activity we will escape from the depressive swamp. But in doing so, we leave the client in their depression. By helping, we continue to spin the depressive whirlpool which pulls the client into a painfully hopeless void. Here we come to the fundamental challenge voiced at the beginning of this book: how to do psychotherapy without helping?

And that's the key! It is precisely because we do not try to help that we are open to yet another way of co-being with the client. By doing so, we also open up another possible way of being for them than just as someone who needs help. So what to do? Nothing. "Do nothing." We get paid for what we do not do. In depression, we do not repeat the relational pattern – we do not save the suffering person. We do not rescue them, even though our powerlessness tempts us to do so. We do not rescue ourselves from feeling powerless. In our experience of powerlessness, we join the other and do not let them suffer alone. We do not help, we do not save, we actively "do nothing."

It needs to be emphasized again that "doing nothing" does not mean not doing anything. "Doing nothing" refers to the inner setting of the therapist, it is the inner work of the therapist with themselves. In that sense, it is not about what we say or how we intervene. We do that as we are used to. An onlooker would, therefore, see normal therapeutic interventions and hear just a normal conversation. It is essential from where we conduct the conversation with the client. We open the space for change not by what we say, but from where we say it. We transform our own way of being with another. As if we are repeatedly reminding ourselves of the choice we are making, how we want to relate to the person in front of us: *"I don't want to be helping you, I want to be with you."* It is about this, our inner setting, not about what

DOI: 10.4324/9781003500148-12

we do. Externally, we can be helping and the client can perceive what we do as help. But we do it from our inner setting, which is free from the demand to help the other.

"Doing nothing" is hard work. It is a very vigorous process of actively deflecting the impulses that draw us into old patterns. We "do nothing," we sit, we listen, we "do nothing." We constantly actively let go of impulses that compel us to do something. How we work cannot be heard or seen. Perhaps it can only be recognized by how much we sweat during such work. After a session we are tired and that tiredness means that we have worked hard. It is hard work. It is alright to be tired, just like we would be after a long, hard journey and now, phew, we have arrived and are resting. We feel fatigue after journeying off the beaten path of habitual patterns.

However, sometimes we are not tired but exhausted. Our exhaustion shows that we have given too much, that we have drawn on personal reserves. That we have given too much because we were trying to help the client to protect ourselves from our own powerlessness. And now we feel exhausted, sorry for ourselves. Okay, that is alright. We got a report that we are investing too much. That's actually interesting: how can we be with another person, how can we really be with them and at the same time invest less? How can we let our encounter alone help? As long as we help, we hinder the encounter. It's a paradox: only when we stop helping can help come through the encounter itself.

We have a meeting with the client in the swamp. Through our own experience, we venture into their territory, we delve into the depressive swamp. We do not stay in our territory where we are strong and safe. We risk ourselves and go where the client is now at home, into the depressive swamp. We break the usual pattern of co-creating depression in a relationship, which tempts us to pull the depressed person out of the swamp, to pull them to us, to solid ground. We hear: *"Nothing has meaning, nothing makes me happy. I have nothing to live for."* And a long, heavy silence. We experience it ourselves and from this experience we answer, for example: *"That must be very hard."* A step into the swamp. We show that we are not afraid of the swamp, that we are willing to venture into it together with the client.

But even that response can be articulated in different ways. And therein lies what is most interesting: where the reaction comes from. From what position, from what setting. We can keep a safe, solidary distance. Something like: *"I can imagine how hard it must be for you."* Or we can allow ourselves to breathe in the heaviness and hopelessness, to experience a dive into the depressive swamp with our own body. We can speak to the client from a position of our own helplessness. Something like:

> *Yes, it must be really hard, I'm feeling it myself right now. And I know I won't pull you out of it now, I have no illusions. I accept the reality of this situation, I am helpless and it is not in my power to help you now. My whole body feels it, it's so hard for me to be helpless.*

We can share an understanding of this when we look into each other's eyes. And we stay. We remain in helplessness with the other. In doing so, we create a bond in which we can sense hope.

It is enough to sit. To sit there and not get in the way. It is about our internal setting, not what we do. Outwardly we can help, but with an internal setting devoid of expectations and the effort to help. We must let go of expectations and be carried by hope. A hope that is materialized in our meeting with the other. Hope is always present in a psychotherapeutic meeting. If there was no hope, we would not be sitting there. But we must not scare it away by pushing it forward; for example, by indicating what could happen. By directing it with our ideas and words. Even by calling it "hope," we scare it away.

By sitting with the client, we send an implicit message: you are worth it to me. You. To me. You are valuable for being. For sitting here. The therapist's presence is the embodiment of hope for the client. It is a healing remedy for the client's experience of their own worthlessness: *"I am useless and it will never be different."*

But how to be present, how to be with the other in such a rare way, when at the same time we do not feel hope in ourselves? It is enough to just sit down. The therapist makes clear by their presence: *"I am sitting here with you, I am devoting time out of my life to meeting you."* Through this, implicitly, with their presence, they make clear: *"I perceive you as a living being that has value in itself. You have value to me, otherwise I wouldn't be sitting here. It's obvious, look, I'm really sitting here."*

Give up and stay. We talked about how to sit with a client. How important it is to let go of expectations, admit helplessness and surrender. To honestly be in helplessness together with the client. If we succeed at this, the battle is far from won. Just the thought that it could be won brings us back to square one. It is a constant process of surrendering – and staying. We notice that we care about the client feeling better (so that we could feel better) – and we let it go, we give up, we admit our helplessness and hopelessness. We stay in it and at the same time we stay there in the situation. With ourselves and with the other person. In depression. Yes, this is alright, this might help. But careful – here are those expectations again, we are once again pushing to relieve ourselves of helplessness. Thus: give up again and surrender to the flow. Like walking consciously and staying present in just this one step, in this moment. And believing that the next step will come by itself, that it will lead us further. And again. And again.

Giving up over and over again, capitulating, admitting helplessness and accepting the reality of the present moment. This is how it is now and that is it. This is how the situation has arranged itself now, this is how it shaped me – that is enough, nothing more is necessary, this is how it is. To dissolve in it, give up yourself, give up the idea of yourself, of your task here, of your uniqueness. And to give up the idea of the other in front of you, give up your good intentions with them. Surrender to the flow of a situation that exceeds us both, to movements we do not understand. To keep the mind in an uncomprehending state. And sensitively, alertly feel presence. Give up and stay and surrender to the concatenation of moments.

Let's now return to Lucie, with whom we opened this book. The psychotherapy session is like an oasis in a desert for her. She's been sinking into depression for years, her husband and sons humiliate her at home, and only here in psychotherapy does she gain some strength. Just enough to get her through the week until the next session. Psychotherapy as support for a system producing psychopathology. Me with her, exhausted, helpless, clueless, without hope for change. This is how we continue therapy for the next two years.

However, I learned one important thing during that time, thanks to my own experience with burnout: it is essential to pay far more attention to myself when working with Lucie. It seems to me like driving a car – it's not enough to just look ahead at the client. Due to the safety risks of psychotherapeutic work, it is also necessary to check the rear-view mirrors, look at myself in the therapy chair from time to time. What experiences of my own appear to me and how do I deal with them? And then I also need to fasten my seat belt in the car, which I think is a nice metaphor for supervision. A supervisor once told me: there is nothing more you can do, hang on. And I took from it: hang on and dial it down. Try to do the same work with the effort reduced to a tenth, set on long-term sustainable fuel consumption.

It started to get interesting. The vicious cycle, the impossibility of making a move in the wider context – Lucie, her family, me with them. And also the vicious cycle in the micro-context of the therapy session: always the same battered weight, the relief of safety, the tearful catharsis and my helplessness. This is how it is, this is what we're spinning in. I don't have to like it, nobody has to like it, but that's the way it is. We need to try not to change it, but rather to just watch it. And to not forget the rear-view mirrors, look in them more often and more carefully – what is happening to me in sessions with Lucie? Interesting thing, I guess I'm starting to get used to the helplessness. Yes, I won't be able to do anything about it. Yes, sometimes it annoys me that I feel quite used. Yes, it is my choice to be here and maybe I will be here like this for another two years. Or twenty...

Everything is still the same, but something has loosened a little in the atmosphere of our sessions with Lucie. It was less of a job for me, more just a talk with her, without any goal or purpose. Professionally frustrating, personally relieving. Why shouldn't I be able to enjoy that oasis too? I reproach myself a little for neglecting Lucie, but she seems to rather appreciate the relief. Yes, I am consciously becoming part of the system, replacing other dysfunctional or missing relationships. I occasionally check seat belts in a supervision and it seems that I am not fundamentally out of the ethical framework of the profession.

Lucie got a puppy from her neighbor. She didn't want it, she was afraid of her husband's reaction. But she was also afraid to reject her neighbor, who needed to get rid of the puppies. The puppy unexpectedly grew into a properly big dog. It slept with Lucie in the kitchen, barked a lot and occupied space, so the men in the household started to avoid the kitchen. Lucie finally had her own place at home. When her husband yelled at her, the dog barked at him even more. Her husband didn't dare to hit her anymore. Time passed and one son moved in with his girlfriend, they had a child. Lucie found herself in the role of grandmother. Her granddaughter loved her and she loved her back.

She timidly suggested whether it wouldn't be enough to meet once every two weeks. Her granddaughter needs babysitting. After some time, she shyly mentioned that she didn't really need psychotherapy that much anymore. After almost five years, psychotherapy gradually somehow faded away. I stopped being important to Lucie, she stopped needing me. She changed, grew older. Even her husband had changed. He had major health problems from drinking, and suddenly he was weaker than her. Life took Lucie to the next stage and she seemed to be doing better. I don't know, I haven't seen her since.

I learned a lot precisely from the simplicity of this story. It just flowed at its slow pace. I was Lucie's support in the lonely part of her journey. I helped her endure. But what helped bring about change was the puppy and the grandchild, not psychotherapy. I feel humbled before the principle of the paradoxical theory of change. When I accepted the situation Lucie and I found ourselves in, change came, albeit in a different way and form than I would have imagined.

Extra-therapeutic factors are responsible for about 40% of the effect of psychotherapy (Lambert, 1992). But even extra-therapeutic factors, such as the dog and the grandchild, are a function of the field's movement. Just like me and my experiencing. When my dismay kicks in and I feel useless as a therapist, I only feel the field movement through myself. Lucie also felt dismayed and useless, and her husband too, probably. My feeling useless is a function of the field movement. I feel it, but it's not me. I'm not a bad therapist, I'm just the therapist that I am. When I say this to myself, I make the fundamental turn. In fact, it's not even me that makes the turn, I was led to it. I heard the intentionality of the field – here, this way is life. This is the way of being of the dog and the granddaughter: we simply are who we are. And they also express it with their love for Lucie. We love you the way you are. When Lucie is able to be with herself like that, she will have a cure for depression.

It is actually simple: the main thing is not to get in the way. To not get in the way with your own efforts. To not get in the way of the change that wants to happen. To constantly surrender, thus clearing the way for change. To open the door for it, to rely on the hope embodied in the meeting and to surrender to hope. Naturally, from clinical experience, a spiritual dimension of psychotherapy opens. Trust in a process that transcends the individual and the relationship and flows meaningfully in its own way. This is a faith that does not have to be tied to religion and culture. Faith that brings inner freedom. We let go of demands on ourselves, and with this released capacity we feed sensitivity and creativity in a depressive situation. We tune in to the movements of the situation and the aesthetics of contact. We listen to the change that wants to happen and that wants to use us to make itself happen.

When we approach it like this, freedom emerges in the depressive situation. And even joy and creativity may crop up through our experience. How? We focus on ourselves again, we work with ourselves. We try to separate the experience of powerlessness from the sense of meaningfulness. We allow ourselves to feel powerlessness, immerse ourselves in it, let it shape us. And at the same time feel the meaningfulness of what is happening. Perhaps sometimes even a quiet joy from the fact that what is supposed to be happening is happening. We are not leaving the client alone, we are not abandoning them, we are with them in depression. This makes sense and we feel the meaningfulness of it in our body.

We thus separate the experience of powerlessness and the experience of meaningfulness so that we can feel them both at the same time. Immerse ourselves into depression and at the same time keep the awareness of our own worth, perceive the hope embodied in the encounter and allow ourselves powerlessness. This is how we are present in a situation, how we bring ourselves into it. Through this, and especially this, the depressive field transforms. We are present differently than how depression shaped us by its pull, because we did not fight it and we let ourselves be pulled in. Through the therapist, the experience of meaningfulness in suffering now appears anew in the depressive field and opens the possibility for the transformation of this field.

Psychotherapy is the art of listening to what wants to be heard. To what is missing. Even in ourselves. Quieting down so we can hear ourselves. Making room in ourselves for what we may hear in a moment and what will transform us. To silence the noises within ourselves by listening to them with curiosity.

If we try to help the client become something they are not, we hinder change. Change will come when we accept the client. We accept the other by accepting everything we experience with them. We accept the other by accepting who we ourselves become in their presence. Change can grow out of our humble, grateful and inquisitive coming to terms with what is. That is enough. Letting go of expectations and sitting in hope.

Bibliography

Lambert, M. J. (1992). Psychotherapy outcome research: Implications for integrative and eclectic therapists. In Norcross, J. C., Goldfried, M. R. (Eds.), *Handbook of psychotherapy integration*. Basic Books, 94–129.

Postscript

Chapter 12

Diagnosis Like the Backrest of a Chair

I'm sitting in front of the client and I'm confused. Something is not right here. We talk to one another, but it's like we're passing by one another. The person in front of me seems to be hearing something a little different than what I'm saying. It's weird. Am I doing something wrong? I'm confused, nervous, I feel anxious. Then I notice that the client is staring into an empty corner. Carefully and with concern, as if there is actually something there. I see. This client may be hallucinating, he could be psychotic. Suddenly it makes sense. We are probably each in a slightly different world. I calm down, lean back in my chair, look at the person in front of me. Now that I don't have to deal with my confusion, I can see him.

A diagnosis helped me make sense of my experience with the client. It's not about describing the person in front of me, I'm not trying to capture how he is dysfunctional. Instead, I use the diagnosis to calm myself down, to not worry about myself, to not be saving myself. As if the diagnosis is supporting, giving me a backrest. And in front of me sits a person whom I now have the capacity to see. The diagnosis helped me see the person. It served its purpose and I can now forget it.

With another client I feel exhausted, impatient, without creativity. I feel incompetent. I drown in these feelings for a while, but then it occurs to me: oh, maybe this client is depressed. Then my experience would make sense. This is how people feel in the presence of a depressed person. I calm down and stop blaming myself. And now I can forget the diagnosis of depression.

By diagnosing the other, I also define my position from where I relate to the other. I may use a diagnosis to create distance. It helps me to better observe the client from afar. And it also protects me personally. Because I am able to say to myself: the client is depressed and I am fine. Then the client and I sit across from each other and there is a diagnosis of depression between us. It protects me and makes the client an object of my care.

On the other hand, I can choose not to protect myself. Then I use diagnostics in a different way. I stop trying to describe the client. I forgo understanding them through a diagnosis. On the contrary, I apply a diagnosis to myself, to my experience with them. A diagnosis helps make sense of my experience when meeting the other.

DOI: 10.4324/9781003500148-14

When I talk about depression, I do not mean that the client has depression. I mean that my experience with another person here and now has the form of a meeting with a depressed person. My mind uses depression to make sense of what I am experiencing right now. In this sense, it is not the content of the diagnosis that is important, but rather the intention with which I use the diagnosis. I am not trying to characterize the person in front of me with the diagnosis of depression. I remain open in how I view the other person and how I will continue to view them.

I may then feel how the diagnosis of depression calms me down, grounds me. Just because I feel incompetent does not mean I am incompetent. It means that I am sitting in a depressive situation that is shaping me in this way. It makes sense to me like this. I lean back on the diagnosis of depression and suddenly I can see the person in front of me. I have more patience for them now. I have more capacity to listen to them. Because the capacity that was previously needed to silence my own insecurity and powerlessness has been freed up.

I also have more capacity to listen to myself. Not to be overwhelmed by the first wave of experiences that washes over me with the client: heaviness, fatigue, helplessness. I am able to not criticize myself for this, to continue to be friendly with myself and accept myself even with these experiences. Accepting the other person then means accepting myself the way I become with the client.

How to deal with a diagnosis? Psychotherapeutic diagnosis (Bartuska et al., 2008) transcends psychiatric diagnostic manuals (such as DSM-V or ICD 10). If we relied only on these manuals in psychotherapy, the risk of manualizing the psychotherapy process would increase and it would limit the authentic contact between client and therapist (Haynes & Williams, 2003). Different psychotherapeutic approaches have therefore developed their own diagnostic systems that correspond to their epistemology and more sensitively describe partial (often relational) events within the psychotherapeutic process. Here, we will focus on the existential humanistic concept of psychotherapeutic diagnosis, which is focused on experience.

We can treat diagnosis as a descriptive and flexible working hypothesis that allows us to connect information from different sources in a meaningful way: what we learn from the client, our observations of the client, observations of our own experience with the client and observations of the relationship arrangement between us and the client.[1] We can also try to observe field phenomena that transcend individuals and their interactions. "In order to understand the dynamics of a process, we must comprehend the totality of a given situation with all its parts and properties" (Lewin, 1935, p. 31).

Therapists who approach clients from the humanistic concept of psychotherapy find themselves in a complex dilemma in clinical conditions. When working with people with more serious mental problems, there is, on the one hand, the uniqueness of the person and their story, and on the other hand, a generalizing psychopathology and diagnosis. Each side has its justification, and by leaning toward only one, the creative tension between them is lost.

When we say words like depression, psychosis or obsessive compulsive disorder, we feel their weight, immobility and also solidity, reliability. And when we say a meeting with a unique human being, we feel a respectful immediacy as well as a disquieting un-anchoring. This is the tension that humanistically oriented psychotherapists need to maintain, even foster, within themselves. It helps us to renew, over and over again, a childlike inquisitive naivety in ourselves and look at the unique being before us. But at the same time, it allows us not to get lost in it all, because we lean on the knowledge and experience of generations of colleagues before us. This tension keeps us creative as therapists. It forces us to remain, in some previously untried way, honest with each client and in each situation with the mentioned dilemma.

If we lean only toward a humanistic perception of uniqueness, we isolate ourselves not only from colleagues who work within the medical system, but also from the accumulated professional experience distilled into the form of diagnostic systems. We also limit the opportunities to meet clients who come to us. There are different kinds of human suffering, and by dealing with them as categories and examining them in this general way, we gain the sensitivity to then more finely distinguish the specific suffering of a particular person and be able to respond to it well. A person suffering from depression needs contact with us that is very different from the contact needed by a person who is suffering, for example, in a borderline way. Thus, if we were to ignore general diagnostic categories, we would be less sensitive to each person's unique needs.

But how can we use the diagnosis so that we do not freeze the live process into a diagnostic box? So that we do not start treating a diagnosis instead of encountering a living person? The key is not to diagnose the person, but a specific kind of experience. We then do not see a depressed person, but we perceive a depressive experience. We simply perceive a person, a human being in its entirety, with which a special kind of experience appears in the moment. We label the experience as depressive based on how we ourselves observe and co-experience it in a situation with the other person. We do not attribute a diagnosis to the person sitting across from us, but we delve into the landscape of their experience, how they experience depression. We can then get a taste for what it is like there.

It is therefore important to realize what we do with a diagnosis within the psychotherapeutic relationship. For example, we can use a diagnosis as a shield to put between ourselves and the client. We will probably be tempted to do this when it is difficult for us to be with the client, when we start to lose ourselves and do not know what to do with our own powerlessness. Then we will probably get relief if we say to ourselves: that person is experiencing something very strange, they probably have some kind of mental disorder. They are psychotic, severely depressed, borderline. And as if we were quietly adding: and I am alright. Such a method of diagnosis protects us, but it also humanly distances us from the client and chills our contact.

Instead of a shield, we can also use a diagnosis as the backrest of a chair. It helps to understand what is happening with us in the presence of the client. Using a diagnosis, we do not label the client in front of us, but with its help we add meaning to our own experience in the situation with the client. When we say "depression," it is as if we mean "I need to sort out what I'm going through with this person right now – and I'm using the concept of depression to do that." This will help us calm down, ground ourselves, stop dealing with our own confusion and stop trying to escape our own powerlessness. It will free the capacity to finally begin to feel the other.

We lean into the diagnosis like into the back of a chair, we leave it behind us. Then we can just as well forget it, so as not to succumb to the temptation to make the constant fresh formation of contact with the client easier. Thus, the diagnosis does not get between us, but remains behind our backs as a source of self-support. We remind ourselves that the diagnosis does not describe the client. A diagnosis describes us, our experience with the client.

Yes, we need to calm down so that we do not have to deal with ourselves and instead have the capacity to perceive the client. But if we calm down too much, if the situation becomes completely clear to us and everything is transparent, we need to be careful. The complex, multi-layered and fluid reality of a meeting of two souls cannot be cramped into a diagnostic category or theoretical conceptualization. It eludes any concept with its uniqueness and unrepeatability. Our overconfidence and calmness suggest that we are missing this elusive reality. If, on the other hand, we do not manage to grasp the situation fully and we are left with a certain unsettling vagueness, we can conclude that we are perhaps on the right track. It is therefore essential to train the ability to endure vagueness in the face of reality, and thus open up to it. To not be paralyzed by the anxiety that naturally arises in an unclear situation. Not to save ourselves, because by doing so we would focus attention on ourselves and cut ourselves off from perceiving reality.

Diagnosis in a Relationship

The use of diagnostics within the therapeutic relationship differs from the use of diagnostics in situations outside the therapeutic relationship. Sufficient distance is needed for clinical diagnosis outside of psychotherapy. A diagnostician deliberately gives up close personal contact with the person in front of them, because such contact would hinder their unbiased assessment. They take the position of an understanding observer who evaluates from a distance. We can imagine that diagnosing dilutes and chills interpersonal contact. This is important for accurate observation and its evaluation. It is as if the diagnostician climbs up to a lookout tower and observes the landscape of the client's experience from that distanced vantage point.

The position of psychotherapists is more complicated, because we have to diagnose within the framework of a therapeutic relationship. As if we are getting into a car together with a client and driving through the landscape of their experience. The distance can no longer be maintained here. This is done intentionally to establish a personal relationship as the strongest effective psychotherapeutic factor (Norcross, 2011). At the beginning of therapy, as joint work begins, a psychotherapeutic relationship develops. Therapist and client enter the therapy process and co-create it. The therapist is therefore counting on the fact that they will not be able to maintain a disinterested distance, and that they will, on the contrary, be very interested in the other person. In psychotherapy, the distance may even disappear completely for a while. These are moments of full I–You contact (Buber, 1937) or moments of meeting (Stern, 2005) in a psychotherapeutic relationship. In such moments, the therapist immerses themselves to the maximum extent in co-existence with the other person, deliberately losing their distance and giving up on orienting themselves in the situation. At the given moment, they do not observe, do not diagnose, but fully experience their existence in the presence of another human being. They meet.

We therapists are both direct participants in a meeting with a client and at the same time reflective observers. It is necessary for us to be able to navigate the therapy process. To do so, we need a certain distance. Yet this does not mean distancing ourselves to the position of an unbiased observer. It is rather as if, in addition to the ability to meet, we are also creating another capacity to concurrently observe. As if we are not changing positions, but rather expanding the possibilities of how we can be in a relationship.

During psychotherapy, we cannot step out of the relationship and become independent observers. Even if we try to, we are doing so within the relational dynamics that we co-create with the client. Our stepping into a safer observer position can then be, for example, avoiding an unpleasant closer contact with those aspects of the client that are difficult for us to accept. And of course the client feels it, reacts to it, the therapeutic relationship transforms and the whole process of psychotherapy modifies. As therapists, we do not even have to say anything diagnostically evaluative, it is enough that we think it. We take a mental distance and the atmosphere of the meeting changes.

Thus, by diagnosing the client, we inevitably diagnose our relationship with them, even at that moment we diagnose ourselves. For example, when we think that a client "is depressed," we evaluate both our mutual relationship and ourselves at the same time. As if we mentally determine our mutual positions: we are the ones who have the power to determine what is healthy and what is not, highlighting the relational asymmetry.

As psychotherapists, we do not give up the ability to phenomenologically observe and gain orientation. However, we are also aware that, as observers, we are also part of the observed. Instead of using objectifying diagnostic criteria, we ask ourselves questions such as: "When I observe depression in a client, how do I feel? How do I contribute to the depression? And what can I learn from this about my relationship with the person sitting across from me?" In this concept, diagnosis becomes an integral part of the entire psychotherapeutic process. We diagnose psychopathology that emerges in a therapeutic situation and we can capture it thanks to our experiencing this situation. Depression emerges here among us. We create it and it creates us. A diagnosis thus becomes the diagnosis of a therapeutic situation, which also includes us therapists.

At the same time, however, we temporarily and consciously step back experientially and observe the therapeutic situation. We thereby create space in us to orient ourselves in the situation. So that we do not merge with it and remain able to meet the other. We gain space to sort through our sensory perceptions, our observations and our experience. We sort and organize them. For a given moment, we add meaning to our experience in the therapeutic process. We use not only our cognitive capacity, but also our informed and cultivated intuition. This entire withdrawal into the observer position can last for a fraction of a second during a therapy session, a few minutes after the end when making notes, or for a longer period, for example during a supervision.

During this withdrawal, we realize that there is a third party present in the psychotherapeutic relationship besides us and the client (Francesetti, Gecele & Roubal, 2013). This third party can be the support of a supervisor, which we remember and draw on during the overwhelming and exhausting work in a depressive situation. Thanks to it, we can anchor ourselves better and remain available to the client. What has a similar anchoring function for the therapeutic relationship is when, as therapists, we recall a certain theoretical model and apply it to our current experience with a client. We create our own theoretical cognitive map (Zinker, 1977), we support ourselves and thus the therapeutic relationship. In this same way, we can relate to the diagnosis as a third party, which remains present in the background, gives a certain framework to the meeting.

Observing and meeting. Remaining in only one of these extreme positions would be unbearable for psychotherapeutic work. Both are necessary for good practice. They are not mutually exclusive, they complement each other. In order to integrate diagnostics into the psychotherapy process, it is necessary to step out of the dichotomous division of "either or" (either we diagnose from a distance or we humanly meet) and instead holistically embrace "that and that." As if we are present with our head and our heart at the same time. The concept of a dynamic relationship between the figure and the background, which are not mutually exclusive but complementary, can help us here. The head and the heart, the observing expert and the engaging human being, are both present at once. Perhaps for a given moment one is more in the foreground, while the other temporarily recedes into the background. They can swap at any moment, one supports the other. Our head and our heart are our body, our body with both of them now sitting in the presence of the other. Perhaps we could say that when observing, we listen to the heart with the head and when meeting we listen to the head with the heart.

Intrinsic and Extrinsic Diagnosis

The psychotherapeutic process can be compared to travelling through a landscape, during which we embark on an adventurous journey together with the client. As therapists, we have a specific role and responsibility. In some phases of therapy we guide the client, in other phases we let ourselves be guided. We travel through a landscape that can be very strange. Together with the client, we discover interesting, useful and threatening features of the landscape we travel. We also often get lost on our way, and then might walk in circles for a while. At such moments, we need to stop and orient ourselves. Take the map out of our backpack and see where the client and I find ourselves. Look around the landscape and compare it with the map. Compare the unique landscape of the client's experience with the general principles of the diagnostic system. If a situation begins to make sense to us, we can give that sense a name, which is a diagnosis. For example, "depression."

With a diagnostic withdrawal, we are not escaping from the relationship with the client, we are just intentionally looking at the map instead of the client for a while. We temporarily shift our focus and support the therapeutic relationship with a third party. As if we were showing the position on the map and clarifying the direction of our common journey. Diagnosis serves as a map in a clinical situation. To be useful, a map must simplify. For that reason, a diagnosis is always simplistic, schematic and does not describe the suffering of a specific person in all its complexity. It helps us orient ourselves, but then we have to be careful to put it back in the backpack. To not wander the landscape with our nose in the map; to not treat the diagnosis.

Diagnosis via a temporary withdrawal can be called *extrinsic diagnosis* (Roubal, Gecele & Francesetti, 2013). It is the result of a comparison between the model of the phenomenon and the phenomenon itself and arises when a therapist consciously focuses on describing the meaning of the given situation. However, when faced with a client, we as therapists cannot always stop, step back and consider how we understand the situation. We usually don't have time for that in a session.

In live dialogue, as therapists we respond immediately. In the blink of an eye, we react with a word, gesture or tone of voice. The important thing is that our reactions do not happen randomly. Here, too, we have clues to help guide our answers. We do not obtain these clues by stepping back and redirecting attention (from the landscape to the map), but on the contrary, by fully immersing ourselves in the flow of the therapeutic situation. We bodily experience our flow in the current of the therapeutic process, which unfolds moment by moment imperceptibly quickly and unpredictably. A different kind of diagnosis helps us here, which enables orientation in the therapeutic situation in a different way.

When we fold the map, we do not randomly start flitting around when meeting with a client. With our sense of orientation, we feel that a certain direction is right. We bodily experience that a certain direction is not to our taste, and another invites us in. Aesthetically, we perceive with our senses where it is good to go and where it is not. With a traumatized client, for example, at a certain moment we feel that it is simply necessary for us to listen and not say anything. We feel the enormous fragility of what they convey. Maybe we are the first person in their life to whom they have opened up, the first they had the courage to finally tell. We do not know. But we clearly feel that it is necessary that we do not intervene in the moment. That we just listen, nod our head slightly and only occasionally make brief eye contact with the client.

A sense of direction guides us where to go, even if we do not necessarily understand why. And then in a few minutes we again feel that now we need to say something. The silence becomes oppressive, stiff and threatens to divide us from each other. We do not know why it is right now, but we feel that there is a need for our voice to be heard in the silence and set off toward the client. A need to invest ourselves. Our sense of direction guides us. This guidance does not come from the outside, from the map, from observing and comparing the landscape with the map. On the contrary, it comes from within, from full immersion in the flow of the situation.

The system of clues that helps us direct our immediate responses in this way can be called an *intrinsic diagnosis* (Francesetti & Gecele, 2009; Roubal, Gecele & Francesetti, 2013). It is based on aesthetic assessment (Joe Lay, in Bloom, 2003) and represents the senses mediated by the perception of the fluidity and grace of what is happening in the now. This implicit knowledge comes directly from the senses. During psychotherapy, it is possible to directly feel elegance, harmony, rhythm, fluidity, intensity and meaningfulness forming the situation into a good shape. Thanks to sensitivity to such an aesthetic criterion, we can also perceive the limitation and deformation of the current contact in the here and now situation, in which something essential is missing. We can sense the suffering that follows and materializes in a co-constructed experience.[2]

Evaluation using an overall aesthetic criterion immediately induces the necessary activity and directs us directly to intervention. Our intervention is then not based on a conscious cognitive consideration of what would be appropriate to do in a given situation. Instead, we perceive the fluidity and grace of what is happening. Or, on the contrary, what is not happening this smoothly. We perceive the situation holistically as an atmosphere (Francesetti & Griffero, 2019), which is, for example, heavy, frozen, tense or fragile. Continuous attuning to the aesthetic qualities of a specific situation directs us by helping us adapt the way we co-exist with the client. However, the guidelines for the next therapeutic step are implicit, we experience them bodily and only in retrospect can we name the process of our decision (e.g.: *"It seemed right to me to do it at that moment"; "I wouldn't dare to say it in that situation"*).

Therefore, even if we do not follow a map, we do not proceed randomly when working with clients. We understand the clinical situation intuitively, and our intuition is cultivated by our reflected experience, psychotherapeutic training and supervision. Intuition guides us through the landscape of the therapeutic situation in its entirety, helping us to orient ourselves through a subtle tangle of signals for which words and concepts are too crude tools.

We compared the extrinsic diagnosis to a map of the landscape and the intrinsic diagnosis to a sense of direction. Both methods serve the therapist for better orientation, albeit each differently. The map provides insight and understanding. The sense of direction is important for immediate next steps in unclear terrain.

Notes

1 When we link these observations into a certain scheme that shows us clues for further work, we follow up the diagnosis with the next step. We create a complex psychotherapeutic *case formulation*, which in Gestalt therapy provides a meaningful holistic picture and guidelines supporting the process of change (Šromová & Roubal, 2022).

2 A therapist perceives the halting of spontaneity as well as the seeds of intentionality and also has the opportunity to contribute to the restoration of the living flow of contact, as discussed in Chapters 6–10.

Bibliography

Bartuska, H., Buchsbaumer, M., Mehta, G., Pawlowsky, G., Wieesnagrotzki, A. (2008). *Psychotherapeutic diagnostics*. Springer.

Bloom, D. J. (2003). Tiger! tiger! burning bright: Aesthetic values as clinical values in Gestalt therapy. In Spagnuolo, M. L., Amendt-Lyon, N. (Eds.), *Creative license: The art of Gestalt therapy*. Springer Verlag.

Buber, M. (1937). *I and thou*. T. and T. Clark.

Francesetti, G., Gecele, M. (2009). A Gestalt therapy perspective on psychopathology and diagnosis. *British Gestalt Journal*, 18(2), 5–20.

Francesetti, G., Griffero, T. (2019). Introduction. In Francesetti, G., Griffero, T. (Eds.), *Neither inside nor outside: Psychopathology and atmospheres*. Cambridge Scholars Publishing, 1–5.

Francesetti, G., Gecele, M., Roubal J. (2013). Gestalt therapy approach to psychopathology. In Francesetti, G., Gecele, M., Roubal, J. (Eds.), *Gestalt therapy in clinical practice: From psychopathology to the aesthetics of contact*. FrancoAngeli, 59–76.

Haynes, N., Williams, A. E. (2003). Case formulation and design of behavioral treatment programs. *European Journal of Psychological Assessment*, 19, 164–174.

Lewin, K. (1935). *A dynamic theory of personality: Selected Papers*. McGraw-Hill.

Norcross, J. C. (2011). *Psychotherapy relationships that work* (2nd ed.). Oxford University Press.

Roubal, J., Gecele, M., Francesetti, G. (2013). Gestalt therapy approach to diagnosis. In Francesetti, G., Gecele, M., Roubal, J. (Eds.), *Gestalt therapy in clinical practice: From psychopathology to the aesthetics of contact*. FrancoAngeli, 79–106.

Šromová, V., Roubal, J. (2020). Case formulation in Gestalt therapy. *Gestalt Review*, 26(1), 63–83.

Stern, D. N. (2005). Intersubjectivity. In Gabbard, G., Person, E., Cooper, A. (Eds.), *The American Psychiatric Publishing textbook of psychoanalysis*. American Psychiatric Publishing, 77–92.

Zinker, J. (1977). *Creative process in Gestalt therapy*. Brunner-Mazel.

Chapter 13

Not Fighting with the Medication

Beginning of a session with Daniel (who was already mentioned in Chapter 4, "Therapists in the Depressive Swamp") after four months of psychotherapy.

Daniel: "Hello."

Therapist: "Hello."

(It seems to me that he looks somewhat spryer today.)

"...How are you?"

"Well, so-so. Actually, it's probably a little better now."

(Well, bless! After those months of hard work, when the depression was not budging.)

"I'm glad."

"Yeah, me too. It was about time... I've slept a little better now. Oh, and I called the job center to see if they had anything for me."

(I wonder what's going on?! He's been plucking up the courage to make that phone call for weeks, we've discussed it over and over again.)

"So you finally went through your fear like we talked about, did you?"

"Yeah, I guess. I don't know, somehow it worked, I just called."

(He probably doesn't want to discuss it, alright.)

"And any results?"

"Nothing much yet, they took my info and said I should ask again later."

(I still think it's a significant step after such a long time. I'll try to explore it further.)

"I wonder how you feel about finally calling."

"Yeah, fine. Actually, it wasn't that bad."

(Oh well. I won't get caught up in it, he doesn't want to go there, I'll stick it out. I'll keep quiet for a moment and see what he offers on his own.)...

"I went to my doctor, a while ago, I forgot to tell you last time."

(He didn't forget, he told me about it. And it took a while before we got to the point that it would be better to have the abdominal pains examined by a general practitioner.)

"Mmm."

"The antidepressants she gave me are good, I guess. Not great, at first, but I don't mind them anymore."

DOI: 10.4324/9781003500148-15

(So that's what it is! He was keeping me in suspense. So the antidepressants started working, that's good.)

"Do you feel better with them?"

"I don't know, maybe a little bit... I also thought that I would start fixing up the apartment my grandmother left me so that I can move out of my parents place again."

(We'd discussed this up and down for several months. He always acknowledged a lot of good reasons to move out from his parents, and it always ended with a "but.")

"Mmm."

"I guess you're right, the drugs helped me. I probably would never have made the move otherwise."

(Like he didn't make a move for a lot of things in his life, right? I didn't want to do the work for him so that he could learn to make moves for himself. He seemed to be getting the hang of having to work on his own to get out of that depressive deadlock he got to in life. I will support him, but I won't do it for him. Like everyone did everything for him all his life. Well, now the drugs have messed things up for us quite nicely. It's nice that he's going to fix up the apartment, that's true. But what's the point of talking about it over and over for months and then a drug just does it for him?)

Medication in the Relationship

When a client uses psychiatric medication, it affects the entire therapeutic situation.[1] Medication changes the course of therapy, intervenes in the therapeutic relationship and affects the results of therapy. It is not just about the pharmacological effect of medication. It is also about how the client experiences medication use. And also how the therapist experiences the client's medication use. As if in addition to us and the client, there was also the medicament in the session with us. Even though the client is using it, the medication also affects us as therapists. It transforms the therapeutic situation and our experience of it. This is probably what we need to orient ourselves in first – how does the client's medication affect us therapists? We have to work on ourselves so that our relationship with the medication does not stand in the way of our meeting the client.

The effect of medication represents a significant external influence, which is usually independent of psychotherapy and the psychotherapist. It can be a difficult situation for the therapist: something interferes with their work with the client and they have no influence over it. But that is not unusual. There are many external independent influences in psychotherapy, and medication is only one of them. Overall, extra-therapeutic factors are thought to be responsible for 40% of the effect of psychotherapy (Lambert, 1992).[2]

Medication can cause a significant shift in a client's experience and behavior. This will be reflected in the therapeutic situation. For example, an antidepressant can help a client mobilize energy and thus significantly influence what happens in a psychotherapy session (as we saw in the example at the beginning of this chapter). Metaphorically, such an influence can be compared to a situation where a client finds a new partner during the course of psychotherapy and falls in love. This external influence, without a direct relationship to psychotherapy, will also significantly affect its course. This client suddenly has options that were not achievable in psychotherapy until then, they feel a surge of energy, believe in their abilities, plan changes in their life. These possibilities appeared without direct connection to the process of psychotherapy. Falling in love opens the way to unsuspected personal potentials, but when it stops affecting the client, the effect can fade. The effect of some medications can be similar, although usually not as dramatic.[3]

Such a significant change in the atmosphere of a psychotherapeutic situation will probably require us therapists to turn to ourselves first. We need to become mindful of our relationship to the medication. A psychotherapist who does not reflect on their attitude and *acts out* their obstinate skepticism and aversion to medication harms their clients to the same extent as a doctor who, when dealing with complex experiential states, focuses only on the psychopathological symptoms, hastily prescribes medication for every discomfort, and thus prevents the natural flow of the psychotherapy process (Fain, Sharon, Moscovici & Schreiber, 2008; Holub, 2010).

The approach to psychiatric medication varies among individual psychotherapists and also develops gradually. It depends very much on the context in which the therapists work and with which clients they work. When clarifying how we relate to a particular medication of a particular client, we can do an experiment for ourselves. We sit the medicament on an empty chair and talk to it, for example: *"Medicament, I'm glad that we complement each other in our work. Thanks to you, I don't have to worry so much about the client."*

Or we can say: *"Medicament, I don't like you. I mind that you are interfering with my therapy. The client thinks he can't do without you, but I'd much rather kick you out of therapy. But I can't because he wants you. I feel powerless, you annoy me. He likes you more than me. He's doing better because of you."*

We may find that we know nothing about the medication and that we need to find out about its properties, become familiar with it, and then continue to explore our relationship with it. But we also need to explore our relationship to medication in general. For example, we may be under the influence of the belief: *"The evidence of well-conducted psychotherapy is that the client no longer needs medication."* We may feel that medication devalues our work and ourselves in the therapeutic role. *"If a client has to take medication, it means I'm not a good enough therapist for them."* Such a competitive attitude toward medication is then necessarily transferred to the relationship with the client and reduces our freedom in our therapeutic role.

Exploring our relationship to medication is likely to open up the topic of our attitude to the medical system, to diagnoses, to psychiatrists. It may be helpful to ask ourselves: *What do I think about psychiatric medications and the psychiatric system in general? Do I or someone close to me have personal experience with psychiatric medications? What is that experience like and how does it affect my attitude toward psychiatric drugs?* The answers to these questions map our pre-understanding, which needs to be consciously bracketed so as not to block the natural flow of contact with a client. There is usually no need to communicate our own attitude to a client. This is our internal work; we need to become mindful of how our attitude to these general issues affects our work with a specific client. Otherwise we risk, for example, projecting our negative attitude toward the medical system onto the medication that the client is taking.

At the same time, however, as therapists, we also need something to hold on to in a situation where our experience of the therapeutic situation is shaken by medication coming onto the scene. We need to create a meaningful framework to make sense of this new situation for ourselves. We anchor ourselves with this and make ourselves available again to meeting the person sitting in front of us in the client's chair. Such a meaningful grasp can be achieved by understanding using a certain theoretical concept, or it is also possible to grasp the situation holistically using a metaphor. Examples of both of these methods are detailed below.

We can understand the use of medication as a certain form of *creative adjustment*, as the best possible way for a client to manage a difficult situation at a given moment. The usage of medication points us to a client's current need. It often performs a support function. It can also emphasize limits and can be used to manipulate the environment. Medication is part of the broader context of a therapeutic situation as well as other external influences affecting a client, such as a job or physical ailments. If a client is more relaxed (or, on the contrary, drowsy) thanks to medication, it transforms the entire therapeutic situation, and the medication thus affects both the therapy process and the therapist themselves.

The introduction of medication into a therapeutic situation may change the therapist's attitude toward the client. When the client is on medication, it can tempt us to relate to the client as an object of treatment, to remain exclusively in the I–it approach (Buber, 1937). Our view of the client might narrow so that the symptoms that change as a result of the medication come to the foreground. Our active work with ourselves then consists of expanding our view of the therapeutic situation. We do not fence ourselves off to symptoms and medication, but include them in a broader concept of our human meeting with the client.

In psychotherapy, we meet a person with a unique story and a unique ability to adapt creatively. Medication belongs in this story. We open ourselves to a human meeting of I–You (Buber, 1937) right here and now with this client and with the entire context of their life, including medication. The client enters the therapeutic situation influenced by a number of external factors: for example, they may be coming off of a sleepless night, a hearty lunch or a morning Prozac. Just as we also come into the therapeutic situation influenced by external factors: for example, we have just finished a strong coffee, had an argument at home last night or just finished an exhausting therapy session with the previous client. Two people meet and their stories intertwine, while psychiatric medication represents one piece in the mosaic of the entire complex situation of their meeting.

Support Along the Way

Medication can be beneficial in the psychotherapy process by facilitating client–therapist contact. Antidepressants, for example, can help reduce immobilizing levels of anxiety in a therapeutic situation. This anxiety is mainly experienced by the client, but it also enters into the therapeutic relationship and is felt by the therapist as well. Energy originally trapped in excessively paralyzing anxiety can then, thanks to medication, be available to the client as excitement (*anxiety to excitement*), enabling spontaneous and meaningful contact with the environment. In the therapeutic situation, we present the environment with which the client can come into contact. Medication can therefore strengthen the therapeutic relationship in this way.

Antidepressants can also act as long-term dampeners of experiences. Clients who take antidepressants describe that it is as if the experiences come to them from a greater distance, with less intensity and acuteness. Medication can thus support desensitization, which is functional at the given moment. The client then does not perceive the feelings of despair and hopelessness so harrowingly. Paradoxically, blunting the intensity of hurtful experiences can help us work with them. For example, it might enable the client to share such "coated" experiences with the therapist and not be left alone with them. In this way, antidepressants help the depressed person to emerge from hopeless loneliness and support a relational experience that breaks the vicious cycle of depression.

When antidepressants began to be used, some psychotherapists refused to combine them with psychotherapy for fear that the medication would obscure important experiences that are the subject of psychotherapy (Holub, 2010). But this attitude is changing, and today the usefulness of combining psychotherapy with pharmacotherapy is supported by research into the genetic and biological effects of psychotherapy, which overcomes the dualistic bifurcation of mind and body (Wright & Hollifield, 2006). Williams and Levitt (2007) also arrive at a holistic approach in their research and abandon the dichotomy of biology versus psychology. The key concept for them is the client's active involvement (*agency*), i.e. their ability to actively participate in the psychotherapy process and make their own decisions in life. Psychotherapy helps the client increase their ability to mobilize their involvement and use the therapist's interventions to gradually learn to heal themselves. Medication is useful if it helps the client to increase their own activity and allows them to be more involved in the psychotherapy process.

In order for us as psychotherapists to get along well with medication, it can help us to think of psychotherapy as a joint expedition. The client is on a journey and the therapist accompanies them. When the client's legs do not work well, they need to lean on a crutch. We can then imagine that an antidepressant supports a person who is deeply depressed so that they can continue to look for a way. Medication does not show the way, but it makes it easier to walk in search of it. This is how we can also look at the combination of psychopharmaceutical drugs and psychotherapy. Medication can serve as a crutch for the client and they can use psychotherapy as a rehabilitation exercise.

The crutch shows us that the person is not able to manage walking without it at the given moment. We realistically see their limitations and their need for external support. But we can also see the crutch as a way for the person to use their remaining potential for movement. This shift in thinking is important: the crutch does not only mean that the client is hitting their limits; that they are limping. It also means that their options are greater with the crutch than without it. The crutch allows the client to use the potential they have left – they can go to work, go shopping, etc. When a client is using medication and a psychotherapist does not want to compete with their effect, the therapist should likely make this shift in thinking. They should view medication as an external support enabling the client to realize their possibilities, which they would not be able to use without the crutch.

Such a metaphorical grasp of the role of medication allows us therapists to meaningfully see our role alongside the effects of medication. We can then compare psychotherapy to a rehabilitation exercise. When a client just leans on a crutch and does not exercise rehabilitation, they are not preparing to walk without the crutch and may remain dependent on it. Or they put the crutch away after some time even without rehabilitation, but then have much more difficulty walking than when, before putting the crutch away, they were rehabilitating and preparing to put the crutch away. In contrast, when a client rehabilitates and then puts the crutch away, they are better prepared to be without it. They can even gain a new awareness of their body thanks to rehabilitation, they can learn to manage it better, gain movement skills and a relationship with their body that they had no semblance of before.

Similarly, a client can manage depression with medication alone. While they are also working psychotherapeutically, they are not only overcoming their current troubles associated with depression. Thanks to psychotherapy, they expand the spectrum of their possibilities in general. They learn to recognize and manage the warning signs of oncoming depression, they learn to use external and internal sources of support, and they may even hear the existential message contained in their depressive experience.

The metaphor of psychotherapy as a rehabilitation exercise and medication as a crutch that can be put aside over time can serve as a framework for us therapists to meaningfully include the effects of medication in our psychotherapeutic work. Such an idea can be helpful to us if the client is using medication, but would like to function without it over time, and this possibility is real. This is a situation where the client on their own comes up with the idea of discontinuing the medication and is willing to endure the discomfort it may bring. They want to actively participate in psychotherapeutic work, they are willing to become mindful of and change their attitudes and make changes in their life. For us and for the client, medication can then be a temporary ally in the psychotherapy process. We can consciously and pragmatically use the alliance with medication and work with it as with other sources of external support, such as the client's stable employment or family background. We help the client consider a good moment to start discontinuing the use of medication. A moment when the client already has enough self-support and other sources of external support. We also help the client examine whether their own potential, which medication allowed them to use, is already achievable even without the medication.

However, there may be a situation where a client with impaired mobility would be able to make another move only with the help of rehabilitation, but they have already gotten used to the crutch. The function of medication has changed; it now serves as a crutch that the client does not want to give up. Medication no longer serves so much as an external support, and instead begins to limit the client's search for new creative ways of adaptation.

The important thing at such a moment is that we as therapists do not push for change. Instead, we can once again lean on a theoretical understanding of the function medication has in the client's life. Medication use is a form of creative adaptation for the client, for example by serving as protection. We therefore respect the function that medication fulfills for the client, and we help the client to become mindful of what the use of medication brings to them and in what way it limits them. Medication can ensure the client's safety, protect them from excessive stress in difficult life situations. But it can also dampen the client's ability to experience and be in contact with other people. We can work with medication as a protective strategy in different ways – appreciate it, confront it, bypass it. We help the client to become mindful of and take responsibility for a balance between receiving external support and relying on one's own resources.

Antidepressants are also beneficial for clients with milder depression. But to work with them, we probably need to create a different framework, a different metaphor. We could imagine that people with milder depression do not need a crutch. They are able to walk without it. But their walk is similar to how Andersen's Little Mermaid walked. She felt pain with every step, as if she was stepping on the blade of a knife. People with milder depression can perceive their experiences with such increased pain. Antidepressants can help dull their perception of this pain – like if the Little Mermaid put on thick-soled shoes. This will allow them to perceive things other than just the pain in their feet, to look around and make contact. As psychotherapists, we then need to find our own meaningful position next to the Little Mermaid.

We probably need to adhere to a different framework when working with people whose severe depression returns in their lives long term. Repeated severe depressive episodes, especially depending on the time of year and without an obvious external impulse, significantly limit the client and may limit some of their abilities in the long term or even for life. Medication in such cases fulfills the function of permanent external support, which the client cannot do without. We can imagine that the medicine here does not serve as a crutch that could be put away over time, but rather can be compared to a prosthesis that replaces a missing limb and allows movement. Such a realistic grasp of the situation can help us come to terms with the medicine and rid us of excessive demands on ourselves and the client. If we had high demands, such as "therapy should aim for discontinuing medication," we would limit ourselves in creative work with the client and could even succumb to the therapeutic nihilism that psychotherapy has no meaning for these clients.

Returning to our metaphor, even for a person with a prosthetic device, rehabilitation has meaning. As a result of the prosthetic, the rest of the body cannot function completely ordinarily. The prosthetic creates various disproportions in the body, different muscle groups are taxed. Rehabilitation can at least partially correct these distortions and the effects of imbalance and thus enable long-term functioning. Similarly, in psychotherapy it is important to help the client to be mindful of and accept the limitations that both the illness and the psychiatric medication present to them. If we, the therapists, come to terms with medication, we also help the client come to terms with the long-term use of medication. Accepting limitations and reducing demands paradoxically opens up space for new possibilities in psychotherapy. What are the possibilities of a joint journey with a prosthetic?

The metaphors describing the role of medication in the psychotherapeutic process presented here can serve as inspiration. However, each therapist probably needs to find their own understanding of what role medication plays in the psychotherapy process with a specific client. Creativity in creating one's own metaphor tailored to a specific therapeutic situation can then help the therapist to free themselves from the demands and expectations that psychiatric medication can awaken in them.

Notes

1 I thank Elena Křivková for her cooperation in developing the materials on which this chapter is based. For those interested in a more detailed elaboration on the topic of the combination of psychopharmacotherapy and Gestalt therapy, I refer you to our joint publication (Roubal & Křivková, 2013).

2 By contrast, specific interventions of a certain psychotherapeutic approach (such as Gestalt therapy) account for only 15% of the psychotherapy effect.

3 The metaphor of falling in love, like any metaphor, has its limits. Being in love enhances experiencing, but also blocks the ability of so-called mentalizing ("love is blind"). On the other hand, psychiatric medication can be expected to modify the client's ability to symbolically grasp their own experience.

Bibliography

Baume, S. (2018). *A line made by walking.* First Mariner Books, p. 42.

Buber, M. (1937). *I and thou.* T. and T. Clark.

Fain, D. S., Sharon, A., Moscovici, L., Schreiber, S. (2008). Psychotropic medication from an object relations theory perspective: An analysis of vignettes from group psychotherapy. *International Journal of Group Psychotherapy,* 58(3), 303–327.

Holub, D. (2010). Kombinace psychoterapie a farmakoterapie. In Vybíral, Z., Roubal, J. (Eds.), *Současná psychoterapie*, Portál, 494–504.

Lambert, M. J. (1992). Psychotherapy outcome research: Implications for integrative and eclectic therapists. In Norcross, J. C., Goldfried, M. R. (Eds.), *Handbook of psychotherapy integration.* Basic Books.

Roubal, J., Křivková, E. (2013). Combination of Gestalt therapy and psychiatric medication. In Francesetti, G., Gecele, M., Roubal, J. (Eds.), *Gestalt therapy in clinical practice: From psychopathology to the aesthetics of contact.* FrancoAngeli, 161–183.

Williams, D. C., Levitt, H. M. (2007). Principles for facilitating agency in psychotherapy. *Psychotherapy Research,* 17(1), 66–82.

Wright, J. H., Hollifield, M. (2006). Combining pharmacotherapy and psychotherapy. *Psychiatric Annals,* 36(5), 302–305.

Chapter 14

Movement in the Suicidal Field

Monika initially came because of fear and anxiety, but as therapy continued, she fell into greater and greater depression. That in itself was disconcerting enough. But I held on to the concept that only now with me, when she is not on her own, can she afford to fall apart and fall downward. It made sense in the context of her life story. Such an understanding helped me to endure with her.

But the depression is deepening and even antidepressants are not helping. Monika does not want to live. In one session, it becomes apparent that the desire to kill herself is so strong that it is becoming predominant. She thinks about suicide often and it is quite thought through. She fundamentally refuses hospitalization because she had an extremely humiliating experience with a psychiatrist years ago. She refuses to expose herself to that again. We keep discussing her situation and the possibilities of how to manage it. I manage to talk her into coming in again next week. I feel relieved – and I try to grab another little piece. Could we schedule sessions for a longer period of time in advance? No. She doesn't want to lie to me and she isn't able to see a future. She simply can't promise that she will be alive for that long.

We've been floundering like this for two months. I feel hopelessness, powerlessness, fear and anxiety. Persuasion from week to week. One supervision after another. Then a text message while I'm travelling for work: "I'm sorry, I know I promised you, but I can't do it. Thank you for everything." First a bit of shock, numbness, then panic starts rising. In this pressure, I have to take at least a moment for myself, to turn my attention to myself. Powerlessness sharpened into urgency, mobilization for action. Okay, switch to the body for a moment, anchor myself in the here and now, breathe, look around. Okay, okay, I'm more composed, I'll call her now. She doesn't answer. I write a message asking her to get back to me. Nothing.

Back to myself again. Consult with a colleague. Realize the ethical dilemma I find myself in. Save a life, act fast, call the police, hospitalization against her will. Hospitalization, which she so fundamentally refuses. For good reasons, I know. She would never trust me again, I would become yet another psychiatrist acting like a jailer. And if she was really 100% determined, she wouldn't have texted me, she just would have killed herself. I'm considering competing values

DOI: 10.4324/9781003500148-16

and can't see any good solutions. But at least it gives me some time and perspective. I text: "I'm so sorry you feel so bad. And I'm counting on seeing you on Monday for therapy, as we agreed." I risk it, but it's on the edge. Two hours of nothing, pretty rough. Then I get a text: "I'll come then."

In half a year, Monika more or less emerges from depression and reflects on this period: "It was terrible. Hopelessness, darkness and terror. I felt like I was drowning, grasping at straws... And it probably wasn't easy for you either, huh?" "Well, it was very hard. The hardest part was that I couldn't do my regular job – psychotherapy. Instead, it was one crisis management after another. I felt like a fireman who keeps putting out a fire for a little moment and then it flares up again. And I put it out again." We look at each other and laugh as we imagine the two metaphors at the same time. The drowning person is grasping at straws and a fireman sprays them with water from the shore. No wonder it took so long.

It's Life or Death Now

We may feel that the atmosphere of the therapeutic situation has changed. Compared to what we are used to in depression, a new, energizing aspect appears in it. As therapists, we experience a strong urgency associated with helplessness and powerlessness. *"Damn, this isn't just talking anymore, it's life or death now. I have to do something about it! But what? I must not make a mistake!"* Here it is fundamentally important that we as therapists do not react immediately to this sense of urgency.

As therapists, meeting a suicidal client can pull the rug out from under our feet and expose our existential doubts. It can disrupt our idea of normal functioning and plunge us into shame and basal self-doubt. Therefore, before we start doing something toward the client, we need to calm ourselves down. We can lean on the general experience of psychotherapists before us. In psychotherapeutic practice, we will encounter suicide regardless of how carefully and responsibly we work (Finzen, 1989, in Rahn & Mahnkopf, 1999). A client thinking about suicide is not our failure or incompetence.

We can also adhere to the theoretical concept of psychopathology, which is co-created in a relationship. Here, the therapist represents the other who participates in shaping the present relationship from which psychopathology arises. The heightened mobilizing urgency and at the same time numbing powerlessness experienced by both the therapist and the client is a manifestation of relationally co-formed psychopathology. It is a manifestation of the suicidal experience that arises between us in the here and now situation (Krysinska, Roubal & Mann, 2022; Mann & Roubal, in press). The suicidal situation has a special dynamic; in addition to the aforementioned urgency, there is a strongly present tendency toward narrowing (Shneidman, 1996). This manifests itself as very limited options at various levels (cognitive, emotional, behavioral, relational).

From the field theory point of view, the therapist's experiences can be understood as an individual manifestation of the processes by which the field organizes. The therapist's experiences of urgency, efforts for control, powerlessness and helplessness belong to the suicidal situation. It is necessary for the therapist to notice them and be able to withstand them, but at the same time not to identify with them. So that they do not blame themselves or the client for how they feel, but that they perceive their experiences as reports on the flow of the current situation that is dragging them along. Accepting this flow and their movement in it allows the therapist to anchor themselves in the reality of the suicidal situation. In the reality of their own experiences, which reveal how excruciating and unbearable it is for the client.

By quieting the sense of urgency, we make at least a little room for exploration in ourselves. We expand by exploring. We do not subject to the dynamics of a suicidal situation that narrows. We also let the client know that we are not afraid to go with them to those domains of their experience from which the further continuation of life seems unbearable. We do not avoid. We do not repeat the avoidance that the client encounters in other relationships. Openly and together with the client, we help bring the scary implicit contents to the surface and give them names. They will then hopefully be less scary and more graspable.

Questions like "do you ever think about killing yourself?" or "Do you ever feel like not putting it off anymore and just killing yourself now?" do not only serve to explore the level of risk, but they also give relational signals: I am not afraid to go into it with you. However, it must be true – we must first find the courage to go through our fear and shame. In this way, we connect experientially to the client, to their fear and shame. Suicide can be understood as a radical expression of extreme shame (Hycner & Jacobs, 1995) driven by the desire to hide forever from the eyes of others. Thus, when we go with a client into experiences of shame, isolation, guilt, despair and worthlessness, on the one hand, we explore areas associated with a higher risk of suicide (Hall, Platt & Hall, 2011). At the same time, we do it with an internal setting: *I want to meet you here too.*

We can thus make room for exploration, first within ourselves and then outside in the therapeutic situation. This will allow us to pick up warning signs that the client is out of their depth, at the end of the road. We try to capture these signs. That is actually what it is all about on a relational level, because these warnings are indirect attempts at contact. We can understand them as a cry: *"Does anyone see that I can't go on anymore?!"* It is an extremely lonely cry. Therefore, the first priority is not to look for a solution, but to listen.[1]

Pre-Suicidal Syndrome

When moving in the urgent suicidal field, the therapist can adhere to special guidelines. The process by which an idea of suicide is gradually born and matures into an act is described as the pre-suicidal syndrome (Ringel, 1973). In order to better manage their experiences in the suicidal field, the therapist can stick to the schematic distinction of three phases of this process (Pöldinger, 1983; Rau et al., 2013). The dynamics of a suicidal situation gradually change, and in each phase the therapist can choose a different strategy both for working with the client and for working with themselves. In principle, we could very simply summarize that in the first phase of contemplation the therapist expands, in the second they balance and in the third they decide. A risk assessment, as described above, helps the therapist to differentiate the individual phases.

In the first phase of **contemplation**, suicidal thoughts arise in the client. Depending on how much the client can consciously handle them, how much they control them, we can judge how far they have gotten in this first phase. At first, suicidal thoughts may bring temporary relief to the client as a way out of a hopeless situation. As the suicidal process progresses, the thoughts become obsessive, bother the client against their will, and they are no longer able to consciously switch to something else. They gradually lose control over them. It then moves from impulses to action. They then move into the second phase of pre-suicidal syndrome.

The contemplation phase is also called a cry for help (Pöldinger, 1983; Rau et al., 2013). It shows us how much the client is suffering in a hopeless situation, how much they need someone to see it. Help here consists of not leaving the client alone in their hopeless situation. Not leaving them experientially because we want to save ourselves from our fear. In the first stage of pre-suicidal syndrome, the task of the therapist is primarily not to panic and to work as usual. Simply explore suicidal thoughts like any other phenomenon that appears in the client's life and that they bring into therapy. The therapist needs to be unafraid to explore suicidal thoughts in the context of the client's life. To not try to solve the client's problems, but together with the client, to look for their meaningful placement in the current situation.

The therapist themselves will most likely perceive the narrowing dynamics of the suicidal field. The important thing is that they do not merge with it, but instead try for expansion instead. First in themselves and then with the client. This then dissolves the urgency of the situation, just as widening banks moderate the force of the current. The therapist expands in themselves by not letting themselves be caught by their worries for the client and by consciously trying to perceive other experiences that arise in the situation with the client. Sadness, pity, mobilization, challenge, shame, helplessness... They expand their view of the client from *"I have to protect this person now"* to *"we will explore this with this person."* The important thing is not to be afraid of your own fear. To go through it. This often manifests itself in words, when we directly name thoughts that are implicitly in the air. We can then ask, for example: *"Do you want to kill yourself to be dead? Or do you want to kill yourself to end life as you live it now?"*

The therapist helps not by protecting the client from suicidal thoughts, but by planting the client's current experience in a wider context, together with the client themselves. And after planting, they study what grows from it. For example, the feeling *"I'm at the end of the road, I can't go on, I have no choice but to kill myself"* becomes *"I'm at the end of the road, I can't go on, I need to go back a bit and think about how to go on."* Or the feeling *"I want to end my life"* becomes *"I want to end my life as I live it now"* and then *"So much is missing in my life and I long for..."*

The second phase of pre-suicidal syndrome can be described as **balancing**. Of those who attempted suicide and did not die, 80% reported in the following two days that they were either glad to have survived or ambivalent about dying (Henriques, Wenzel, Brown & Beck, 2005). This ambivalence is also a guide for the therapist. The client is balancing and so is the therapist. The client physically experiences the urge to die, which manifests itself, for example, in impulses to jump out of a window or under a truck on the street. They gradually lose control over them, they become compulsive. The client is balancing on the edge between life and death. And the therapist tries not to leave them alone in it. They need to balance as well. They provide space for the client to talk about both competing tendencies. About the force that pulls them toward death, which is clearly expressed physically in suicidal impulses; and also about the force that pulls them toward life, which is rather hidden, but actually clearly visible in the fact that the client continues psychotherapy.

The therapist will probably naturally be tempted to fight for life. However, this is a subtle trap into which the client's loved ones fall. When the therapist takes the side of life exclusively, the client is left with only the remaining polarity, the side of death. The more the therapist tries to fight for life, the more the client will accent death. They will try to make the therapist really see how strong the power toward death is. The original internal balancing of the client can thus be externalized in the therapeutic relationship. If the therapist sees life as the only option and only pushes the client to life, paradoxically, the risk of the client actually attempting suicide can increase. The client feels misunderstood and abandoned in their suffering.

For this reason, it is necessary for the therapist to first balance within themselves. To admit that the tendency to live and the tendency to die make up the client's experiential reality at this moment. To admit that each of these two tendencies has its weight and its reasons, that both represent a real possibility for the future. Yes, the client can live on and they can also end their life. Suicide is one of the options that people have (Hillman, 2013). This is a reality that the therapist needs to internally take into account and give space to when they start working with a suicidal client.

Further, the therapist can be guided by the fact that the client's basic need is to feel understood (Bion, 1962). The therapist themselves experiences an uncomfortable, unsettling ambivalence, and it is precisely through that that they can connect experientially to the client. Now, they can both experience it together and the client may not feel so abandoned in their existential struggle. They may experience relief: *"Yes, finally someone really sees what I live in and does not try to convince me that it should be different."* By working on themselves, the therapist creates a space in which the client feels accepted with what they are experiencing. With their confusion and ambivalence.

Part of the therapist's balancing is a sense of responsibility. The therapist needs to consider how much responsibility in a given situation they take for the therapy process and also for what happens with the client next. The more the pre-suicidal syndrome progresses and the client loses control over suicidal impulses, the more there is a need for the therapist to provide a firmer framework for the client's existential struggle. This framework can create a more structured psychotherapy session, including a plan of next steps. It can also consist of external support in the form of a diagnostic assessment by a psychiatrist, the use of psychiatric medication or hospitalization as a form of protecting the client from uncontrollable suicidal impulses.

It is important that we maintain the basic attitude of *creative indifference* (Friedlaender, 1918) during these security measures, in which we do not fight exclusively for life. Instead, we try to convey to the client the feeling that they are accepted as they are now, with both death and life tendencies. Within ourselves, we are balancing on a narrow ridge (Buber, 1937): we want to answer, on the one hand, the need for a technical approach, for exploring risks and creating strategies, and on the other hand, the call for human contact. Due to this, we can maintain balance within the relationship with the client (Howdin & Reeves, 2009) between thoroughly examining the risk with a derived strategy of therapeutic approach (relating at the level of I-it) (Buber, 1937) and creating a space for a meeting with another human being (relating at the I–You level) (Buber, 1937).

The third phase of pre-suicidal syndrome is characterized by **deciding**. It can be confusing for the therapist that the client is suddenly calmer and more relaxed. They freed themselves from the unbearable tension between the opposing forces of death and life by choosing death. If they have really decided, they have no reason to come back to therapy. So we only meet clients in this phase if they are brought there by someone else, for example their close ones. Here, the therapist decides whether to take responsibility and make a choice for the client, usually considering hospitalization. The ethical dilemma that was already present in the previous phase of balancing becomes more acute: two opposing values compete inside us and there is no absolutely correct solution. On the one hand, we feel a professional responsibility, because we see the client's situation in a wider context. On the other hand, we respect the client's freedom and the unique direction of their story. If we decide to take responsibility for the client, our internal setting with which we make this decision will again be important. So that it is not a decision just out of fear, but also out of concern for the client as a person: *"I want to give us a chance to meet again in the future."*

Note

1 Hillman (2013) even claims that trying to prevent suicide in psychotherapy does not help. That instead of prevention, it is essential to validate the client's human experience.

Bibliography

Bion, W. R. (1962). *Learning from experience*. Maresfield Reprints.
Buber, M. (1937). *I and thou*. T. and T. Clark.
Christensen, L. S. (2013). *The half brother*. Arcade, s. 288.
Finzen, A. (1989). *Suizidprophylaxe be psychishen Störungen*. Bonn.
Friedlaender, S. (1918/2013). *Schöpferische Indifferenz*. Gesammelte Schriften Vol. 10. BoDBooks on Demand.
Hall, R., Platt, D. (1999). Suicide risk assessment: A review of risk factors for suicide in 100 patients who made severe suicide attempts: Evaluation of suicide risk in a time of managed care. *Science Direct*, 40(1), 18–27.

Henriques, G., Wenzel, A., Brown, G. K., Beck, A. T. (2005). Suicide attempter's reaction to survival as a risk factor for eventual suicide. *American Journal of Psychiatry*, 162, 2180–2182.

Hillman, J. (2013). *Suicide and the soul*. Spring Publications.

Howdin, J., Reeves, A. (2009). In the fragility of contact: Working with suicide risk in the dialogic relationship. *British Gestalt Journal*, 18(1), 10.

Hycner, R., Jacobs, L. (1995) *The healing relationship in Gestalt therapy – a dialogic/self psychology approach*. Gestalt Journal Press.

Krysinska, K., Roubal, J., Mann, D. (2022). A safe place for Katie: A Gestalt therapy perspective on her suicidal experience. In Gunn, J. F., Lester, D. (Eds.), *Perspectives on a young woman's suicide: A study of a diary*. Routledge, 109–123.

Mann, D., Roubal, J. (in press). Gestalt therapy approach to suicide and self-injury. In Bohall, G., Bautista-Bohall, M. J., Musson, S. (Eds.), *Dangerous behaviors in clinical and forensic psychology*. Springer.

Pöldinger, W. (1983). *Die Abschätzung der Suizidalität*. Huber.

Rahn, E., Mahnkopf, A. (1999). *Lehrbuch Psychiatrie für Studium und Beruf*. Verlag.

Rau, T., Plener, P., Kliemann, A., Fegert, J. M., Allroggen, M. (2013). Suicidality among medical students: A practical guide for staff members in medical schools. *GMS Zeitschrift für Medizinische Ausbildung*, 30(4). doi: 10.3205/zma000891.

Ringel, E. (1973). *The pre-suicidal syndrome. Psychiatria Fennica*, 209–211.

Shneidman, E. (1996). *The suicidal mind*. Oxford University Press.

Index